D1496106

Medical Saints

For David Murray

With best wishes +
thanks for your
wonderful daughter

Jackie Duffin

25 Nov 2013

MEDICAL SAINTS

Cosmas and Damian in a Postmodern World

———◦◦◦———

JACALYN DUFFIN

OXFORD
UNIVERSITY PRESS

OXFORD
UNIVERSITY PRESS

Oxford University Press is a department of the University of Oxford.
It furthers the University's objective of excellence in research,
scholarship, and education by publishing worldwide.

Oxford   New York
Auckland   Cape Town   Dar es Salaam   Hong Kong   Karachi
Kuala Lumpur   Madrid   Melbourne   Mexico City   Nairobi
New Delhi   Shanghai   Taipei   Toronto

With offices in
Argentina   Austria   Brazil   Chile   Czech Republic   France   Greece
Guatemala   Hungary   Italy   Japan   Poland   Portugal   Singapore
South Korea   Switzerland   Thailand   Turkey   Ukraine   Vietnam

Oxford is a registered trade mark of Oxford University Press
in the UK and certain other countries.

Published in the United States of America by
Oxford University Press
198 Madison Avenue, New York, NY 10016

Library of Congress Cataloging-in-Publication Data
Duffin, Jacalyn.
Medical saints: Cosmas and Damian in a postmodern world /Jacalyn Duffin.
pages cm
Includes bibliographical references and index.
ISBN 978-0-19-974317-9 (hardcover: alk. paper) 1. Spiritual healing—
Christianity. 2. Miracles. 3. Medicine—Religious aspects—Catholic Church.
4. Cosmas, Saint—Cult. 5. Damian, Saint, d. ca. 303—Cult. 6. Christian saints.
I. Title.
BT732.5.D835   2013
231.7'3—dc23   2012034143

Photos by the author unless credited otherwise.

1 3 5 7 9 8 6 4 2

Printed in the United States of America
on acid-free paper

For
Ross Duffin
Bert Hansen
Anita Johnston
and
Ana Cecilia Rodríguez de Romo

Contents

List of Illustrations   ix

List of Tables   xi

Acknowledgments   xiii

Prologue   xv

1. Medical Miracle   3

2. Doctor Twins: from Cyrrhus to Toronto   31

3. Talking to Pilgrims in the New World   61

4. Chasing Saints in the Old World   97

5. Miracles, Medicine, and MEDLINE   137

6. Conclusion: Home to the Clinic   165

Epilogue   175

Tables   179

Notes   189

Bibliography   201

Index   221

List of Illustrations

1.1	Auer rods inside a leukemia blast cell	5
1.2	La *miraculée* going to the Vatican, December 1990	18
1.3	Cosmas and Damien receiving a trousse of medical wisdom from God	21
1.4	Roman Forum with Basilica and Castor and Pollux Temple	24
1.5	Pope John Paul II, Père Bouchaud, author, and Dr. Jeanne Drouin	28
2.1	Poster for Toronto feast	32
2.2	Fra Angelico, The Healing of Palladia	34
2.3	Fra Angelico, Cosmas and Damian and their Brothers crucified	35
2.4	Fra Angelico, The Decapitation of Cosmas and Damian and their brothers	35
2.5	Fra Angelico, The Miracle of the Black Leg	38
2.6	Basilica of Saints Cosmas and Damian and San Lorenzo in Miranda, Rome	42
2.7	Crowd at the Toronto feast, 1992	48
2.8	Procession with Toronto Hospital in distance, 2010	49
2.9	Boys dressed as the saints, Utica, 1996	55
3.1	Toronto procession on College Street, 1998	67
3.2	Devoted parishioner, Utica, 2003	68
3.3	Joe DeCandia carrying his saints, Howard Beach, 1999	78
4.1	Statues of the santi medici, Naro, Sicily, 2001	106
4.2	Hospice and sanctuary to santi medici, Riace, Calabria, Italy, 2001	108
4.3	Wax votives for sale, Riace, Calabria, Italy, 2001	109

4.4   Ceiling painting, San Cosma Albanese,
      Calabria, Italy   110
4.5   Daytime procession, Alberobello, Puglia, 2001   114
4.6   Women *cavalieri* carrying the statues,
      Alberobello, Puglia, 2001   115
4.7   Saints Cosmas and Damian Basilica,
      prayer card, Bitonto, Puglia   118
4.8   Sanctuary to the medical saints, Ravello,
      Campania, 2001   124
4.9   Wedding in cathedral with santi medici,
      Isernia, Molise, 2001   127
5.1   Change in Medical Publishing on
      Religion, 1965–2009   142
5.2   Dance of the Giglio, capo and lifters,
      Williamsburg, Brooklyn, 2003   146
5.3   Ceiling painting, Conshocken, PA, circa 1960   147
5.4   Procession leaving church, Conshohocken, PA, 2005   148
5.5   Cosmas and Damian as Marassa in Montreal, 2002   151
5.6   Marassa based on Cosmas and Damian in Haiti, 1993   152
5.7   Catalan goigs, Barcelona, 1961   156
5.8   Statues of William and Charles Mayo,
      brothers and physicians   157
5.9   Cover of the 2010 program for the American
      Osler Society   159
6.1   Visit to the patient. Jean Chièze, 1942   168

List of Tables

1 Responses: What are your origins?
How far have you come today?   179

2 Responses: Is it important to you
that the saints are twins? Doctors?   180

3 Responses: Why do you attend the feast?   180

4 Responses: Have you attended other
feast-day celebrations? Where?   181

5 Responses: Do you know of any miracles?   181

6 Summary of Miracles following appeals to
SS Cosmas and Damian as told by pilgrims   181

7 Towns with shrines dedicated to the medical
saints in Puglia   184

8 Doctor saints   185

Acknowledgments

OVER THE COURSE of twenty years, this project has incurred many debts. Nearly three hundred anonymous people participated in the surveys. I deeply appreciate their cheerful willingness, pithy candor, and insights, all of which were crucial to this study.

For their generous descriptions of local traditions and personal experiences, I am deeply grateful to Thérèse Beaulieu, Michele Burke, Giuseppe Cannito, Mary Colonardi, Joseph and Clara DeCandia, Sal DiDomenico, Sr., Sal DiDomenico, Jr., Deacon William Dischiavo, Beatrice Gruttaroti, Ersilia Janetta, Anthony Leccese, George Minisci, Mary Moïse, Lise Normand, Natale Persico, Eulalie Riopel, Giovanni and Lorita Sisto, Silvio the chef, Dan Tomaselli, Yolette Toussaint, and Renzo Valilà.

Support also came from members of religious orders who welcomed the project and patiently answered questions. In particular, I thank Sister Marguerite Letourneau of Montreal; Father William Woestman of Ottawa; Father Ralph Paonessa, Father Gregory, and Father Stefano of Toronto; Father Albert Gardy of Philadelphia; the late Father Francis J. Evans of Howard Beach; Father Gaspar Genuardi of Conshohocken; Father Thomas V. Doyle of Brooklyn; Brother Mark McBride of Rome; and Madre Sonia Sapena of Valencia, Spain.

Challenging conversations with friends, family, and colleagues influenced the writing in myriad ways. It is a pleasure to recognize their contributions—some from long ago and others very recent—Patrick Bellegarde-Smith, Peggy Brown, Brian Chung, Marcella Damiano, Heike Drotbohm, Jeanne Drouin, the late Gina Feldberg, François and Martine Gallouin, Marijke Gijswijt-Hofstra, Joseph Goering, Monica Green, Francesco Guardiani, William Helfand, Frank Huisman, Franca Iacovetta, the late Pierre Julien, the late Tom Keebles, the late Ross Kilpatrick, Olga Kits, Kristine Krafts, Anne Leahy, Joseph Lella, Beth Linker, Joshua Lipton-Duffin, Jennifer Macleod, Gilles Maloney, Sheila McCullough, Michael McVaugh, Joseph Merrill, Margarita xiv Acknowledgments

Mooney, Lois Myers, Anne Overell, Ann Pollack, Paul Potter, Carlos Prado, Chantal Regnault, Ira Rezak, Guenther Risse, the late Charles Roland, Terrie Romano, Monica Sandor, Max and Rosita Shein, Giulio Silano, Sergio Sismondo, Ineke van Wetering, Adrian Wilson, Jessica Duffin Wolfe, and Cherrilyn Yalin. I also acknowledge the sobering stimulus of colleagues who disapproved of the work.

Many librarians and archivists also contributed to this book—in particular, Joseph Coen of the Diocese of Brooklyn, Anne Smithers, Suzanne Maranda, and the stalwart members of our Interlibrary Loan team at Bracken Health Sciences Library, Queen's University, and the remarkable *signori* of the Vatican Secret Archives reading room.

Valuable research assistance came from Ian Billingsley, Blair Ernst, and especially Julia Cataudella and Rachel Elder. Beyond gathering data, their enthusiasm, insights, and questions helped to shape the final product.

Two research grants from the former Hannah Institute of the History of Medicine of Associated Medical Services, Toronto, supported travel to Europe and research in the Vatican Secrets Archives and Library. In addition, I heartily thank Queen's University not only for its sustaining system of sabbatical years—no fewer than three of which went into this project—but also for the privilege of working in the tonic atmosphere generated by its open-minded students and faculty.

At Oxford University Press, I was fortunate to find editor Cynthia Read, whose confidence, wisdom, and efficiency transformed the bleakest of outlooks into energy and optimism. Earlier portions of three chapters appeared in the magazine *Saturday Night*, December 1997, and in two conference volumes from St. Michael's College, University of Toronto, both edited by Joseph Goering, Francesco Guardiani, and Giulio Silano, *Saints and the Sacred* (2000), p. 11–24 and *Mystics, Visions, and Miracles* (2002), p. 149–160. I thank the editors for permission to use these materials.

Yet again Robert David Wolfe deserves a paragraph of his own—handling logistics, making meals, finding miracles, turning phrases, negotiating Italian byways, reading churches, newspapers, and endless drafts, spending holidays hopping from one obscure hamlet to the next, waiting uncomplainingly for closed doors to open, and remaining ever vigilant for signs of "the boys," with whom this quasi-Catholic of a nonobservant Jew has quietly accepted to live for most of our marriage.

Finally and hopefully fittingly, this book on brothers is dedicated with thanks and admiration to my siblings, both biological and spiritual: Ross Duffin, Bert Hansen, Anita Johnston, and Ana Cecilia de Romo. Without them, it would not exist.

Prologue

THIS BOOK WAS many years in the making, partly because it took a long time to gather the information, and partly because—having begun to drown in data—I did not know how to organize it.

Sparked by an unusual event that I had lived in my life as a hematologist, it evolved into a quirky, two-decade-long quest to answer questions that I asked as a historian. Had Jeanne Drouin never invited me to read a set of bone marrows back in 1987, I might never have wondered what Saints Cosmas and Damian were doing in Toronto. And I might never have noticed that they, or any other physicians, had ever become saints.

As the possible answers to the historical questions accumulated over the years of study, it seemed that any narrative on the topic could find no good place to start, and no good place to end. Some sources stretched far back into remote protohistory—others emerged from the present, which soon turned into the future, relative to the moment when the questions arose. Indeed, on some level this project is endless. The way out of the dilemma was shown by my musicologist brother, Ross. He reminded me that stories are the best part.

History is about the present as well as the past, and it is also about ourselves. We tend to hide our personal experiences in writing history. But the questions, subjects, and strategies stem from our own time, while the interpretations belong to our proclivities as individuals. The chronology of this book, therefore, is the chronology of the project; it is autobiographical.

So in addition to explaining historically and medically what medical saints may be doing in our time, this book is also about the origins, methods, and growth of a research project—a little history of a history. Springing from curiosity, it proclaims the vital significance of the literature, but also of colleagues, friends, and those shadowy "peers." The acknowledgments are much more than pro forma; they are the real bibliography.

Medical Saints

I

Medical Miracle

*I call a miracle anything which appears arduous or unusual
beyond the expectations or understanding of the one who
marvels at it.*
—AUGUSTINE OF HIPPO, *De utilitate credendi, 16, 34*

NO MISTAKING IT. A speck of dark red in a malevolent sea of deep blue
with just a trace of green. I dropped a bead of oil on the slide and turned the
microscope up to high power. There it was. An Auer rod, the eponymic term
for a minute particle inside a human blood cell. It nestled beside the pale,
mauve nucleus of its strange, evil-looking cell—one of many similar shapes
swimming in the thin smear of an unknown patient's blood. The particle
proclaimed its home to be a "blast" cell, diagnostic of acute myelogenous
leukemia, the most aggressive human malignancy. Average survival without
treatment was two-and-a-half months; with treatment, two years—at best.

Grim news for the patient, it was true, but waves of relief spilled over me.
This slide was only the first of a hundred or more left to read, and already I
had a diagnosis. The samples were all taken from the same individual on
several occasions during 1978–79. The other slides of blood and bone
marrow waited in cardboard trays beside me. It would take nearly seven
hours over a couple of days to complete the reading—low power and scan,
medium power and identify, high power only if necessary. The process felt
like an examination.

In a way I *was* being tested. It was April 1987. I had been a hematologist for
eight years, but unforeseen events interrupted my career. After certification in
internal medicine and blood diseases, I had moved with my nephrologist husband and our three-year-old son to Thunder Bay in northern Ontario. My
husband, age thirty-three, was the town's only kidney doctor; at thirty, I was
its first specialist in blood. We quickly developed large consulting practices
and happily embraced our role as "pillars of the community" so generously

offered by the multicultural town. On the first anniversary of our arrival, he was cycling to work and hit by a truck; he died minutes later.

I stayed in Thunder Bay for a time, with support of friends, colleagues, and patients, but there came an amazing opportunity for a new life and marriage with David, an old friend. My son and I joined him in Paris where he was serving as a Canadian diplomat. Armed with letters from former professors, I went to the big hematology centers of Paris looking for work, or at least a chance to do research. Nothing. Oh they were polite. I could go back to medical school if I wanted; I could translate their articles for publication (which, sometimes, I did); I could help in the operating room as a scrub nurse during a strike (at which I failed miserably on my only attempt). But I could not see patients, except by straining from the back of the crowd surrounding the professor on his rounds. He—always a "he," a tall "he"—would lean forward from the germy, outer environment and wave to the frightened, sexless, hairless person tied to tubes and wires inside the plastic life island. "Ça va?" the professor would ask, smiling and waving; and then, he would move on, not waiting for the reply.

I couldn't stand it. My new husband was an important person and worked long days in Canada's mission at the Organization for Economic Cooperation and Development. My son went to a Parisian public school and quickly acquired superior French and a sense of shame over his mother's accent. They both were busy and I was at loose ends. After a long search for something edifying in the hospitals, I found medical history and Professor Mirko Grmek, who became my advisor and gave me direction with a fascinating project. Just before our return to Canada in mid-1985, I had successfully defended a doctoral thesis about the invention of the stethoscope. During the public examination in an upper room of the Sorbonne, I kept wanting to laugh. It seemed too improbable that I—blood-doctor from Thunder Bay—would be arguing in French with three cultivated gentlemen about angels on the head of a pin. I wanted to go back to hematology.

After returning to Canada, I hung around the Ottawa General Hospital's hematology service for about a year. The doctors were friendly, but they had no vacancies. I went to rounds and tried to speak without saying anything stupid. I volunteered to cover the ward at Christmas, and I did a little consulting in Hull on the Quebec side of the river. One hematologist claimed to be looking for someone who could do "wet lab" research, but he hired a fresh graduate with no more "wet lab" experience than I. Of course, I couldn't really blame him. The young man may have *wanted* to do "wet lab"; I wanted patients, people, their histories, and the elegance of the clinical workup. Only eight years after my certification and notwithstanding my large practice in Thunder Bay not so long ago, I was fast becoming a "has-been." This marrow-reading of leukemia was a test of my credibility.

Dr. Jeanne Drouin, one of the hematologists at Ottawa General Hospital, made it happen by asking if I would look at "a few" marrows for an "independent expert opinion." My new friend agreeably conversed with me in her first language, though her English far outclassed my French. We were about the same age and she was sensitive to my being out-of-work in contrast to her "arrived" position as a university professor. She seemed almost apologetic about the request, as if she were offering scut work. The rules of the situation required that she provide no information at all about the case and that I write a report about the blood and marrow. I would be paid the usual consultation fee, of course. Any further facts about the case were elusive for the time being. Perhaps someday I might find out the rest.

I leapt at the chance, but immediately began to worry. It had to be for a lawsuit, I reasoned. What if I failed? What if I missed the subtleties in the diagnosis that had obviously called the case into question? Perhaps I would be summoned to court and the lawyers would mock my credentials: a historian more than a doctor masquerading as an "expert." I had to get it right or risk embarrassing Jeanne's confidence in me.

But that Auer rod made the diagnosis on the first slide (Figure 1.1). Surely something more mysterious had to be lurking there to explain the need for an investigation? The diagnosis was so obvious, and the disease, so deadly. True to her word, Jeanne had provided no information. But the slides revealed some secrets anyway: the patient had been admitted to the Ottawa General—these were our slides with our patient numbers. The little dumbbell shapes of

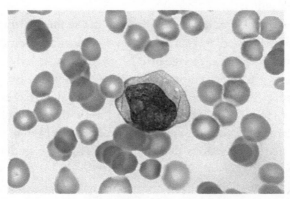

FIGURE 1.1 Auer rods inside a leukemia blast cell. Photo courtesy of Dr. Kristine Krafts.

inactivated X-chromosomal material on the nuclei of normal white blood cells told me that the patient was a woman. She had almost no blood platelets, the cells that help to make clots. I imagined that she would have been covered in bruises and petechiae—little blood spots—and that she may also have had a fever. She would be frightened. The initials "L. N." and the dates were scratched in pencil on each slide. Fourteen different bone marrow samples had been taken between April 1978 and May 1979. Her doctors had been concerned.

With those dates and that diagnosis, she must be dead by now, more than eight years later. Her uncomprehending and grieving family was probably suing the physician for malpractice—a rather unusual occurrence in Canadian hematology, but not impossible to imagine, especially since the advent of bone marrow transplants around the time of her illness had increased the possibility of cure.

The second set of slides indicated that the patient had received some chemotherapy. The marrow, which had been packed with leukemia cells at her admission, was now depleted. The remaining cells were broken with changes in shape and development that were probably the result of drugs. A few more marrows, a few more weeks, and she was in remission. Yay!

The remission was easy to diagnose by following the rules: the presence of only normal elements in the blood and mostly normal-looking cells in the marrow with no more than 5 percent leukemic blast cells. Because I had not been given the laboratory reports, I was counting the cells "by hand"—one hundred on each blood film; five hundred in each marrow—using a mechanical counter like a typewriter with a different key for every type of white blood cell. When the total reached one hundred, a little bell made a satisfying "brrring," just like the tiny, toy cash register I had played with as a child. I was thirty-six. How old had this poor woman been? Had she lived as long as I? I began to feel guilty.

Remission, remission, it went on through the summer of 1978—but the doctor had been worried or skeptical, because a bone marrow was done every month. Would such invasive vigilance be given to an elderly patient? She must have been young. Four months after the remission, the blast cells in the marrow crept up over 5 percent and by the following month they were circulating in the blood. Relapse. Oh dear. Now I knew that she had to be dead. Back in the late 1970s, the only cures in this disease had been in patients who were maintained in continuous, first remission. Relapse meant that her disease was incurable.

More treatment seemed to follow, the marrow was emptied again, and it was a long time before healthy cells reappeared. But they did come back with normal blood, while marrow blast cells stayed under 5 percent. Hooray! Remission again. Hematological lore says that second remissions are always more difficult to achieve and maintain; and they are usually shorter. In my brief experience, I had never known this rule to be contradicted. The first remission had lasted only four months; would this one last as long as four weeks?

Only a few more slides were left to examine. Remission with continuing treatment effect—I could imagine the patient was by now taking daily chemotherapy pills as maintenance therapy, and perhaps regular injections too. Would the last slide show relapse? Probably. No, it didn't. More remission with more evidence of treatment. The end.

Ah. I saw it now. She must have died of what is called "therapeutic misadventure." After a hard-won second remission, her doctor had been trying to keep her blood stable with ongoing chemotherapy, and during that treatment she died, probably of an infection. In leukemia, infectious complications were common, because of the disease and because of its treatment. I felt sorry for the physician and pondered the failure of communication that would allow a family to think that the doctor could be blamed for this death, which had come one year later than if nature had taken its course.

I went back over all the slides and grew confident in the diagnosis and the evolution of the disease. Nevertheless, I took care to insert many disclaimers in the report, pointing out that none of the information normally used to indicate a blood diagnosis had been provided. I wrote: "I was given no clinical details . . . no machine blood counts . . . no special stains for cell types"; "I do not know if or when the patient was treated . . ." and better, for some hypothetical, future cross-examination by an aggressive lawyer, I asked, "Has the patient been treated?"

I submitted the report to Dr. Drouin for forwarding to the parties who had requested it. A few days later, I bumped into her in the hospital corridor. She seemed pleased with me and told me that she had agreed with my assessment. Relief. I had passed the unstated test. But what about the case? "Is it malpractice?" I asked, "or . . ." Perhaps it was Jeanne's relaxed smile that made me continue, "or are we dealing with a miracle?" "C'est un miracle," she replied. The patient—her patient—was still alive all these years later! And my report? It had been sent to the Vatican. A few weeks later, the consultation fee was duly paid by check drawn on the account of the Grey Nuns of Montreal.

A miracle?! It was *remarkable*, certainly, that L. N. should be alive in a second remission that was so much longer than the first. But scarcely ten years had passed since her diagnosis. I would hesitate to call this a cure. She could relapse at any minute, and I for one would not be surprised. And how could it be a miracle if she had been treated by the standard methods of the time? Over coffee, Jeanne explained.

In April 1978, Lise Normand was in her late twenties and single when she turned up in the emergency room covered in bruises and feeling weak. She was heavyset, but otherwise healthy looking. Her acute leukemia was diagnosed right away. The chemotherapy made her suffer greatly. She vomited—and back then our management of drug-induced nausea had not been as effective as it is now. She lost her hair and developed fever. Her remission lasted such a short time. Jeanne remembered how depressed the team felt on recognizing the relapse. The side effects of her new treatments were worse than before, with jaundice and excruciatingly sensitive mouth sores. Lise nearly gave up hope. But when she finally went into remission a second time, her strength improved. Jeanne decided to keep her on maintenance therapy for as long as Lise would tolerate it. She did not expect her patient to survive the year.

But at the end of that first year, Lise was well, and she wanted to stop her drugs. Jeanne cautioned that the situation was precarious. Why alter something that seemed to be working? Lise followed the advice for three more years, but as she entered the fourth year of her second remission, she flatly refused to carry on. She confessed that she had been skipping doses, because she felt herself to be cured. Jeanne was worried, but had to admit that there were no rules to follow at this point. So few patients had survived in a lengthy second remission; and, those drugs were poisons: sometimes they were thought to cause second malignancies. With reluctance, she agreed to stopping the treatment.

Then, Lise Normand told her surprised physician the rest of the story. During her relapse, she had been visited by her aunt, a Grey Nun from Montreal, who gave her a medal with the image of the order's founder, Mère Marguerite d'Youville. Lise's friends and family had been praying for her recovery since the onset of her illness, but it was only during her relapse that they suggested she turn to Mère d'Youville. Suddenly, she knew that this was what she must do. "Why not?" she said to herself, and from that moment on, she was comforted by the spiritual presence of the blessed founder. Lise believed that Jeanne had been chosen as the instrument of her cure; it was her duty to carry on with the treatment as long as her doctor recommended, testing her all the time for the day when the drugs could finally be stopped.

Jeanne told me that the story had been "toute une nouvelle"—a complete revelation to her. After their years of struggle together, she thought

that she knew this patient very well. Yet here was an event of great importance that had taken place long ago to fully permeate her patient's experience of their shared journey. A practicing Catholic, the doctor had been
raised in a large family within a French Canadian community like that of
her patient. Jeanne could not simply ignore or discount what her patient
was saying, nor could she ignore her training as a physician-scientist; she
had other beliefs too. She asked that Lise stay in touch; come for regular
check-ups, just in case. Lise agreed, partly, she made it clear, out of a sense
of gratitude.

But Lise had not finished with surprises for her doctor. She asked that her
medical records be submitted to the Vatican. For many years, the Grey Nuns
had been pursuing the cause for canonization of Marguerite d'Youville. Just as
the diagnosis of leukemia followed a precise set of rules, detecting sanctity
also had its rules. An exemplary life documented by a careful biography was
the first step. In order for Mère d'Youville to be recognized as a saint, her
beatification in 1959 had to be followed by at least one new "miracle." The
nuns believed that Lise's case could provide the necessary step for the first
Canadian-born saint.

Miracles have a precise definition and meaning in the process of making
saints. Only God can bring about events contrary to nature; a miracle wrought
by appeal to a deceased human being is a sign that the soul is with God. The
rules for diagnosing a miracle were laid out in the late sixteenth-century
Counter Reformation, and formalized in the 1730s by Prospero Lambertini,
who became Pope Benedict XIV.[1] First, an event must be attributed to the
intercession of the candidate for sainthood. Second, no scientific or material
explanation can account for the event. Third, both the original appeal to the
would-be saint and the event must have been documented, and the records
submitted as evidence to a local tribunal. Fourth, independent witnesses must
attend the tribunal and agree that the event cannot be explained by existing
science. Finally, the entire case and the testimony of witnesses must pass the
careful scrutiny of a Vatican committee of specialist physicians. As part of the
final step, the "postulants," or ambassadors of the cause, must counter all objections raised by the office of the Promoter of the Faith, who is also known
popularly as the "Devil's Advocate."

In answer to her patient's request, Jeanne transmitted the documents. The
second remission was only a few years old and the doctor would not have
been surprised if the Vatican committees decided that the submission was
premature. But when the response of the medical advisory board was announced a few months later, she was completely taken aback.

Instead of finding the case premature, the doctors in Rome disputed Jeanne's reading of the marrows and her management of the case. Yes, they agreed, the diagnosis was acute myelogenous leukemia, but there had never been a second remission, they said. The marrows, which she (and later I) had read as the first remission, were not remission. Leukemia cells were there all along, the Italian doctors argued; in finding a remission, we had simply succumbed to wishful thinking. The second round of treatment given four months after diagnosis was just what was needed to bring about a good, solid, "first" remission. Prolonged first remission was possible in 1 to 5 percent of cases. The case was "fortunate," yes; but a miracle? No.

The nuns were disappointed. Jeanne was understandably annoyed, and having been caught in the same so-called "error," I grew indignant on her behalf. We had both followed the rules for diagnosing a remission, and with no prior knowledge, my readings matched hers. In the heat of the clinical moment, with a half-treated patient lying bald, febrile, and vulnerable to bleeding and infection, time and the "retrospectoscope" were unimaginable luxuries. That was why we relied on rules for reading bone marrows. With no inkling of the process, I began to see where I fit in.

Realizing that Dr. Drouin had her own reasons for dismay, the nuns asked if the slides could be reviewed by an independent witness. A hematologist in central Canada was apprised of the situation and offered to do the readings. But he waffled and refused to argue with the Vatican committee. Now the nuns were annoyed too. The clinical scenario was not reproduced if expert doctors were provided with all the details of the case, including its unusual outcome, before they looked at the slides. A physician must be found who would be willing to spend all that time reading the marrows without being told a thing. Who better than an unemployed but not overly ripe hematologist looking to prove her worth? Me.

The disclaimers with which I had peppered my report as a talisman against an imagined, legal interrogation had unintentionally contributed to the cause of the Grey Nuns. My hand-counted differentials on each marrow sample naïvely but loudly supported the time-honored, hematological rules with numbers: a first remission; a relapse; and then a second remission. Unlike me, the good doctors on the Vatican committee knew that the patient was still alive; they had been caught discounting hematological evidence, second-guessing, reinterpreting the facts with a hindsight that would have been impossible clinically and should have been forbidden technically. Their interpretation had been colored by Lise Normand's extraordinary survival, which they found difficult to believe.

What a high. No wonder Jeanne was pleased. It was definitely the most unusual case I had ever seen. I didn't expect much more. These things obviously take time. Dr. Drouin left for sabbatical in France and I was invited to look after her practice. Sometime during her absence, I was contacted by the Grey Nuns. They thanked me for my help and expressed their hope that my report—and its unwitting "I-know-nothing" tone—would cause the Vatican committee to reconsider. Soon we learned that the case was to be reopened for examination as the final miracle in the dossier of Marie-Marguerite d'Youville, now well on her way to becoming the first Canadian-born saint.

The nuns made an appointment to visit my office. I was uncomfortable. Reading marrows I could do, and sending my work elsewhere did not trouble me at all, provided that the patient had agreed. But I am not a Catholic and, though raised a Protestant, I could not claim to be religious. Twice I had married Jews. Best stick to hematology. What could they possibly want?

Two intelligent, forthright women in simple, knee-length habits greeted me like an old friend and told me how much my cooperation had meant to their cause. My angst deepened. I reminded them that they had paid the going rate for that cooperation. They conceded the point. But now, they said, more of my time was needed and payment was out of the question. The rules of making saints required that an ecclesiastical tribunal be held on the case of Lise Normand to which all supporting characters must be willing to testify voluntarily. A bishop would preside; a canon lawyer would be present. I could be paid for the consultation, but not for testimony. Witnesses must not appear to be bought.

Quickly, I said that as much as I had been impressed with the happy outcome in the case, I could not possibly testify to a miracle. No, no, they said. That would not be necessary. The Vatican would decide about the miracle. I would continue to be the expert witness. It was simple: first I must recognize my own report; second, I must tell the tribunal if the outcome could be explained by science.

This task was plausible—just. I weakened. "You see," they continued, "we have reason to believe that Mère d'Youville has interceded several times for sick people. But medical cooperation is difficult to obtain." Last year a little boy was cured of a dreadful immune disease (after a marrow transplant, it was true), but his pediatrician refused to testify before a tribunal, and the case could not be used.

"My husband is Jewish," I said. Surely now I would be disqualified. "Fine, fine," they said, looking absolutely delighted with my life choices that contrasted so starkly with their own. Even better in many ways, they implied, because my situation would indicate that I had no vested interest in the outcome

of the saintly process. Nor did I need to worry about speaking to a "lay audience" made up of "clerics": a Catholic doctor would be present as a friend
of the court to interpret my words should I say something in "medical-ese"
that could not be understood by the bishop and the canon lawyer.

Who could resist the opportunity to participate in the canonization of
her country's first saint? The nuns were not asking me to make a statement of
faith. They were asking me to be a hematologist—something I had been
wanting people to ask of me for several years. I wondered about the pediatrician who had refused to cooperate. Was it fear that had kept her silent in the
face of her patient's request? What could testimony have appeared to cost?
Did one risk conversion? Could there actually be any experienced doctors left
who thought that people got better simply and only because of what we do to
them biologically? On the other hand, I was pleased: had that pediatrician
agreed, I would have missed this incredible adventure.

A summons to a tribunal seemed to demand authoritative preparation. I
reviewed the medical literature and photocopied the most recent articles on
survival rates in acute myelogenous leukemia of adults, highlighting in bright
pink relevant passages on relapse and shorter durations of second remissions.[2]
My claims about remissions and survival were not isolated; they would rely
on observations of the most respected hematologists in the world. In nervous
moments, I could easily find and quote the pink passages.

Before the meeting, I was asked to read Lise's own statement. She wrote
in simple, moving words of her experience with illness and her astonishment
at the mystery of what she clearly believed to be her cure. The word "cure"
troubled me.

The tribunal met over two days in early December 1987 in a large room of
Saint Paul University, an Ottawa seminary. They would hear from Lise, her
friends and family, Dr. Drouin home from sabbatical, and me; we were invited at different times. At the long head table, Monsignor Morin presided;
Father William H, Woestman, a professor at Saint Paul University, served as
the canon lawyer; and Dr. Pierre-Paul Allard was the medical friend of the
court. Several Grey Nuns were seated at the side as reporters and witnesses.
The atmosphere was strangely formal, but the welcome was warm. I took my
place at a small table equipped with a microphone connected to a tape-
recorder that would register my testimony.

After the introductions, I was required to recognize my typed report on
the fourteen bone marrows taken from Lise and to confirm that I really had
been given no prior information about the case. The investigators then asked
if I had a scientific explanation for the "cure"? The constant repetition of the

word "cure" was irritating. In medicine, I explained, we make predictions only by statistics. We can find aspects of the case that correspond to favorable prognostic factors, such as the patient's age, sex, and genetic markers on cells. I showed how some features of this case had pointed to a long survival; other tests, developed since Lise had been sick, might also have generated more information had they been available at the time. Then I produced the photocopied articles to show that the rare patients who appeared to have been cured of this disease were almost always in *first* remission. Only in extremely rare cases did a second remission outlast a first, and I was not aware of a "cure" in a second remission after the kind of treatment used for Lise. The members of the tribunal received the photocopies gratefully and added them to their files. They then asked how many other patients I knew like Lise; I knew of none in my own experience or in the literature.

The committee seemed pleased with my answers and ready to let me go, but, perhaps as a requirement, they asked if I had anything else to say about the case or the process. I had not expected that question, but their sincerity and obvious desire that I say all I could as a hematologist made me respond. "Yes. I am uncomfortable with your use of the word 'cure.'" Absolute silence. Had I thrown cold water over their hopes and ambitions? With difficulty, I continued. "Lise could develop leukemia again. Only a few years have passed since her diagnosis; she is still young, and all my training teaches that her case should be incurable. What happens if you make a new saint on the basis of this "cure," and then she has a relapse? I wouldn't be surprised, but what happens to you and your cause? Is it no longer a miracle? Would the canonization be revoked? Are you prepared to wait out the many more years of Lise's natural lifetime until she dies of something else?"

The investigators looked crestfallen. But this reality check was precisely what they had needed me to do. Finally, I felt some affinity for those doctors in Rome who must be bombarded with the hopes of postulants convinced that their heroes are worthy saints. I imagined hundreds of people caught up in the thorny rules that demanded "proof" of miracles in order to capture the church's recognition of something they believe to be obvious and true. What made up the miracles in the late twentieth century? Were they only medical? Must all miracles now be sanctioned by doctors? How could a self-respecting church tolerate this incursion of skeptical scientists onto their spiritual turf?

The cruel words had been spoken and recorded. Embarrassment followed for us all. Dr. Allard broke the silence. "But she has had eight years of life without symptoms or signs of any disease!" Partly out of a medical desire to soothe and make amends for the terrible objections I had just raised, partly out of trying to be polite, I babbled. "I don't know the rules." I then heard myself saying, "do you need to use the word 'cure' in order to make claims for a miracle? After all, we are all going to die some day. If no other patients are like Lise, who has enjoyed almost a decade of unexpected health, could that not be seen as a miracle in itself? Instead of 'cure,' maybe could you call it a 'miraculously' prolonged second remission? If that's possible."

I was beginning to hope for the potential saint, for the unknown patient motivated to repay a perceived blessing, for the aspirations of the gentle sisters in the room, and for the good clerics who sat opposite trying so hard not to be duped by the seductive process that had led to our improbable encounter. But it couldn't be helped. I continued in the hematological vein, "Sometimes when a leukemia returns, after chemotherapy or after a bone marrow transplant, we are able to use special tests to show that the new leukemia cells are different from the old ones. We refer to it as a 'second' leukemia, and treat it as a 'new' and different disease." Now I was launched on draconian predictions. "When she relapses, perhaps you might be able to say she had been 'cured' of the 'old' leukemia and that the final episode was due to something else?" I finished lamely.

The mood improved a little. "A prolonged second remission," the assembly repeated. Heads nodded. I cheered up. They were not angry with the sobering message; possibly it was a challenge. I flattered myself that they could now rewrite their proposal in a fashion that might prove more convincing in the eyes of those naturally skeptical hematologists in Rome whose medical expectations, like mine, had made them reject the case as a miracle once already. And my hematological integrity remained intact. If they were to reject the case again, it would have to be for the right reasons and not for an unfair revision of the rules of pathological diagnosis.

I was excused. In the lobby waited the sisters who had come to my office and Dr. Drouin who had already testified. Lise had gone home. We were joined by members of the tribunal including Father Woestman. They were ebullient; the tensions were melting into celebration. The earlier testimony of the patient had been exciting and surprising. Apparently, her prayer to Mère d'Youville had been echoed not only by her aunt, but by several Ottawa valley parishes that had registered novenas on the same day, at the same time. We contemplated the reverberations of a thousand good wishes floating up to the blessed foundress in heaven. Was combined prayer actually louder?

"Hey" I turned to Jeanne, "we could do a randomized, double-blind, controlled trial on how many novenas it takes to make a miracle." She grinned, but nudged me to shut up; the nuns burst out laughing. Father Woestman said that the whole business of miracles was under review and that someday a person might be recognized as a saint for their life and deeds alone. Until the process changed, miracles were required by those rules of canonization set down in the eighteenth century. "But what moves me," he said, and he was visibly and happily moved, "is that today is a great day—a great day for women: the patient is a woman, the attending physician is a woman, the expert witness is a woman, the postulants are all woman, and the saint herself is a woman, and . . ." he paused to emphasize the full impact of what was coming, "they are all Canadian!"

Silly it seemed, but tears started anyway. We went our separate ways marveling at the remarkable morning. That evening the sisters who had acted as court reporters came to my house with a typed transcript of my testimony. They asked me to read it carefully and to correct any potential mistakes, especially in the medical words. I was to initial each page and each correction. My two children danced around. As the night was cold, we invited the nuns to come inside, but they declined politely and waited outside in their car with the engine running. There were very few mistakes. A sister came inside to collect her precious document.

She thanked me again and asked permission to offer the children ballpoint pens with the image of the prospective saint and a color cartoon book of her life history. "Of course," I replied, poorly concealing my amusement at the chattels of advertising. The sister drew herself up with a smile and said, "You know, it isn't for the splashiness of the miracles that we want her to be recognized as a saint. We are looking for the miracles because we must—the rules require it. But it is the example of her life that we want to spread. When her sanctity is widely acknowledged, others will learn about her and draw strength and comfort from her as a role model." That night I read about the life of Marguerite d'Youville and decided that it was time to investigate more about her and the business of saints.

Jeanne gave me a copy of the authoritative biography that had been published in 1945 by historian Albertine Ferland-Angers in preparing the cause for beatification.[3] It was satisfyingly full of footnotes with references to archival papers. Marie-Marguerite du Frost de Lajemmerais (widow d'Youville) was born in 1701 at Varennes on the south shore of the Saint Lawrence River near Montreal. She led an ordinary life, went to school, married, and had six babies of whom only two survived, both boys destined to become priests. Her marriage was unhappy—"an apprenticeship in suffering," the author said.[4] Her husband was an unscrupulous trader who supplied the native peoples with cheap alcohol in exchange for valuable furs. He, and apparently also his mother, had abused his wife, but Mère d'Youville accepted her lot with equanimity. She even nursed him patiently through his last illness in 1730. After his death, she began to care for the sick and disabled, first a blind woman, then many more. Mère d'Youville was joined by other devout women in founding the Sisters of Charity of Montreal, the Grey Nuns. So many people came to depend on their help that a large building was needed. She appealed to the city of Montreal and, in 1747, was given the right to occupy the dilapidated but still beautiful "General Hospital," erected by the Frères Charon in the previous century. Under her direction, it became a soup kitchen, a hospice, and a refuge for children, battered women, prostitutes, and the sick. Quebec was conquered by Britain in 1759; in the ensuing strife, the sisters bestowed their charity equally on all, English or French. Mère d'Youville died in her bed after a long illness, bravely borne, in 1771.

During the nineteenth century, the sisters founded new chapters, hospitals, and schools in Ottawa, Winnipeg, the Canadian north, and other countries. The epithet "Grey Nun" came from the pejorative French term *grisette*, meaning a drunken streetwalker; the citizens of Montreal had used it to mock the widowed women and their charges, who were not virgins. The sisters adopted the insult as their name out of humility and as a reminder of their origins.

I began to think of the thousands of documented miracles that must reside in the Vatican archives. I imagined a history project on these stories—suspecting that the prominence of medicine in the decision-making process must have been recent. Father Woestman responded to my queries by sending copies of Prospero Lambertini's rules on canonization. He also supplied many other references and sources of information about the making of saints.

In April 1988, five months after the tribunal, Monsignor Morin called. Would I meet Lise Normand and then return to him to explain whether or not the encounter would alter my previous testimony? I had never met the woman who had suffered leukemia, although her story and her bone marrow were familiar. She came to the clinic where we sat awkwardly discussing her remarkably good health, her work, and her small aches and pains. She was big, blond, rosy-cheeked, and shy; her eyes sparkled and her whole demeanor exuded vitality. The blood counts were entirely normal. At the seminary, I reported that my statement did not need changing. Monsignor Morin took me to lunch in the cafeteria, where I tried to tell him how I was intrigued with the untapped historical potential of the miracle cases in Rome. He listened politely as young seminarians smiled and stole glances our way.

Months went by. One clinic day, an intelligent, elderly woman with chronic leukemia came for her checkup. She had never made a secret of her religious devotion. Her son, my friend and colleague, had been headed for the priesthood before he turned in another direction for medicine and a wife. The patient was well, but inclined to fret about the frustrating lack of control over her frightening but asymptomatic condition.

"What should I eat? What do I wear? What can I do?" she persisted. Her condition must not be a burden, I explained. She was free to eat, dress, and do as she pleased. After we had been over the same ground a few times, I said she might try praying to Mère d'Youville. She paused and an ironic look crept into her eyes.

"Will that really help?"

I shrugged and, thinking of my Jewish father-in-law, replied, "I don't know, but it can't hurt." I never made that recommendation to anyone else before or since. Patients might seek healing in a multiplicity of ways, but they do not go to the doctor for spiritual advice.

We all waited. I accepted a position at Queen's University as historian in the medical school where I continue to do a little hematology. Occasionally I would hear from one of the sisters. Each Christmas, the Grey Nuns sent a card with their blessings and wishes for a healthy new year.

In 1990, I devoured the new book *Making Saints*, by Kenneth L. Woodward. Religion editor of *Newsweek*, Woodward seemed to have written just for me. Using examples of recent causes, interviews, and a thorough examination of the documents, he explained the rules of canonization, also describing the medical committee and the role of "Devil's Advocate," whose responsibility it was to raise all possible refutations. Paul VI had hesitated to make new saints, but John Paul II was dealing with the backlog of causes in a revitalizing flurry of saint-making. Saints reflected their cultures, as did their miracles. Marguerite d'Youville fit the role model that the church sought in a saint for the 1990s: a woman (slightly unusual), who had been unhappily married (more unusual), born in Canada (a first).

Mère d'Youville had a rival for the honor of being the first Canadian-born saint: Alfred Bessette, known as Frère André, an illiterate thaumaturge who died in 1937 and had been beatified in 1982. Frère André inspired the building of Montreal's Oratoire Saint Joseph, where his preserved heart can still be seen in an eerily lit red coffer, surrounded by hundreds of crutches and braces left by those who believed themselves cured through his intercession. Miracles would not be lacking in his case, but he might be too recent or "conventional" by saintly standards. Based on Woodward, his cause seemed less likely to succeed in the climate of finding saints to fit the times.

Finally, in October 1990, the front pages of English and French dailies announced that Mère d'Youville would be canonized on December 9, 1990; the case of Lise Normand had been recognized as a miracle (Figure 1.2). Phone calls came from Dr. Drouin and the nuns to make sure I had been paying attention. I asked if the miraculous healing was considered a "cure" or a "prolonged second remission," but they did not know; these

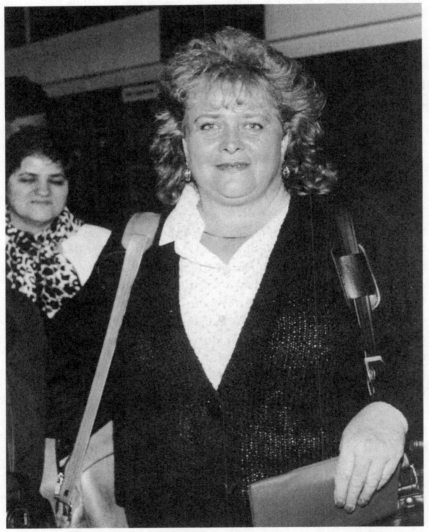

FIGURE 1.2 La *miraculée*, Lise Normand, going to the Vatican, Photo by John Kenney, *Toronto Star*, December 9, 1990.

details no longer mattered. Posters arrived from "Exotik Tours" offering three different package-tours to Rome, with or without side trips to the Holy Land and Lourdes. Then I received a personal letter from Marguerite Letourneau, Mother Superior of the Sisters of Charity, and an invitation to the canonization. The nuns were offering to pay my round-trip, economy fare as a token of gratitude for my unpaid appearances before Monsignor Morin.

My first reaction was that I could not possibly go. It seemed wrong to accept the gift. Perhaps it was intrusive for a nonbeliever to attend such a special ceremony. "Nonsense," Jeanne told me over the phone. She was going; she wouldn't miss it. "If the nuns didn't want you, they would not have invited you," she said. "You were part of the journey and they want to celebrate with all those who contributed. You should receive their invitation as an honor, because that is how it is intended. If you accept, they will view your presence as mark of esteem. It will show that you respect their cause, even if you do not 'believe' in it."

When I accepted, I asked if I could bring along my husband at our own expense, even if he could not attend the ceremony. As Jeanne had predicted, their prompt reply assured me that I had made the right decision, and they invited David to attend the ceremony.

It was crazy to leave just as term was wrapping up—even for a week. But shorter flights were prohibitively expensive. My mother came to stay with our children; a graduate student volunteered to help. David packed many books, which he planned to study each night in preparation for his doctoral examinations in political studies, scheduled for right after our return. We would arrive a week before the event, rent a car, and travel a little, ending our explorations in Rome with the canonization. I made a list of the medical-history sites in Italy that I had always wanted to see.

The flight was long. A white-knuckle flyer at best, I kept having problems with my ears. As the plane drifted downward, my eardrum was fit to burst. A kind-looking woman, seated a row or two ahead, looked back a few times with sympathy while tears ran down my cheeks.

Upon arrival, against all predictions, our rented car was ready, the weather was clear, and my ears popped. We set out for Ostia Antica, the ancient port of Rome and the first site on our list. Having walked the archeological ruins, we headed to a bakery to pick up lunch. It was one o'clock in the afternoon.

Ten minutes later, we discovered the locked trunk of our rented car had been forced open and everything inside was gone—our suitcases, clothes, winter coats, camera, return tickets, and all the books, including David's political science texts and Woodward's *Making Saints*. We still had our passports and a credit card; everything else had vanished. We gazed around; the empty windows and streets mocked our foolishness. A police report would be needed and we were sent on to a nearby town. Ironically, the only Canadian we knew in Rome was a government physician, the former priest son of Jeanne's elderly patient. He came the eighteen miles to our rescue, bringing an Italian translator who helped to compose the long list of items stolen. I began to mourn for my most cherished clothes, gifts from David and the children that I had planned to wear on the big day at Saint Peter's Basilica.

I wanted to go straight home. David said that we should press on at least for one night to regain our composure. We took the car back to the airport expecting to be chastised. The officials merely grunted, did not even look at the damage, and gave us another vehicle—identical to the first. We found a miserable hotel by the side of the autoroute, and called home to describe our trauma and find out what was happening. They were sorry for us, but sounded fine. The temperature plummeted and we slept poorly, clinging to each other in the same clothes we had been wearing since we left home.

In the morning, we decided to stay. We had almost nothing else to lose. I worried about David's not studying for the big examinations. He said that he would cram when we returned. Near Florence, the Irish nuns at Fiesole were expecting us. On learning of our predicament, they sent us scurrying down the hill to Standa—Italy's answer to Woolworth's—where our immediate needs of underwear, toothbrushes, soap, and towels could be filled before closing time.

Traveling with nothing but a little car had its advantages. No pictures to be taken. No bags to carry. No real reason to lock the car, although we did. Nothing to do but keep moving, walking, looking, and eating anywhere that would accept a credit card. The memory of that journey is filled with exquisite tenderness. Orvieto, Florence, Siena, San Gimignano, Bologna, Padua, Venice, Ravenna, Urbino, Assisi. In Padua, the ancient medical faculty, *Il Bo*, was closed. But our hotelier made several calls describing me grandly as a "professoressa di storia de la medicina," and we were given a private tour of the sixteenth-century anatomical amphitheater, Galileo's lectern, and William Harvey's crest. We searched the nearby Euganean Hills for the supposed site of the background scenery for the "muscle men" in Andreas Vesalius's great anatomical atlas of 1543. In the Scrovegni Chapel we saw the frescoes of Giotto, the story of saints Anne and Joachim, parents of the Virgin.

Saints were everywhere. Florence boasted many celebrated images of martyr saints Cosmas and Damian, twin brothers who were also medical doctors (Figure 1.3). From my historical reading, I knew that they were patrons of medicine, surgery, and pharmacy. Because the powerful Medici family took the *santi medici* (medical saints) as their patrons, they appeared in works of great artists who enjoyed Medici sponsorship. Padua had been high on my medical history list, but we realized it was far more popular as a destination for pilgrims devoted to Saint Anthony, patron of those seeking lost objects. His tomb was festooned with the leavings of the faithful, evidence of more miracles. And in Ravenna despite an inescapable, bone-penetrating cold, we found mosaics of many saints, including Cosmas and Damian again, but also the famous emperor and his wife rendered in holy postures. Saints could be political.

The heavy traveling had been hard. It was time to head for Rome and the reason for our enforced holiday. We drove west out of Urbino headed for Assisi on the other side of the Apennine Mountains. As we climbed, it began to snow. A simple problem for Canadians, we thought, but our little rented car was not equipped for the weather, nor were any of the other vehicles slithering over the narrow, winding road. Ice and poor visibility brought us to halt;

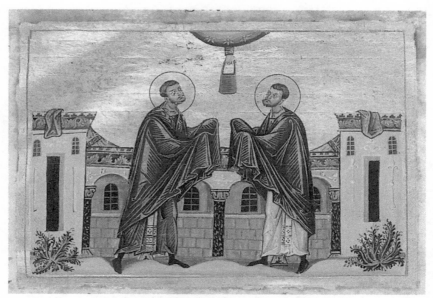

FIGURE 1.3 Cosmas and Damien receiving a trousse of medical wisdom from God. The *Menologium of Basil II*, 12th century. MS Gr. 1613 Biblioteca Apostolica Vaticana.

we waited for two long hours at the side of the road as darkness and more snow fell steadily. We crept back a mile or two to a gas station with a restaurant. The place was packed; fifty or more truck drivers, smoking, drinking, and eating through their wait until the end of the storm. I was the only woman. There was nothing to read. We ordered a big meal and ate it slowly. A radio reported that this storm was the worst in many years. Around one o'clock in the morning, the owner offered us his bed, and we accepted instantly. The room was frigid, but we lay close in our dirty rumpled clothes with muscles clenched too tight to shiver, grateful to have escaped the thick smoke.

I could not sleep. Here we were, Canadians with no coats trapped in the Italian mountains by winter. This embarrassing predicament meant that we might not reach Rome in time for the canonization. And what about our flight home? The stolen airline tickets still had to be reissued. Maybe we would be here for weeks.

The futility and stupidity of our situation washed over me again and again. I thought about the many strange occurrences that had brought me to this improbable low. The patient, her serious disease, the miraculous "cure," the strange rules for making saints, the nuns, my vain hope of returning to life as a real hematologist that made me accept the offer of the marrow readings in the first place. Then there was my own widowhood that had lead me to that desperation. Of course, Marguerite d'Youville had been widowed too, and I had to admit that she had suffered far more than I, in marriage and in life. Right now I was probably passing the chilliest night of my life, but she had felt at least this cold on many occasions. She and her sisters must have been freezing on the winter night in 1765 when their hospital burned, destroying ten years of hard labor in a few hours. As the nuns were bemoaning their loss, the reverend mother told them to kneel and thank God for the wonderful opportunity to start over again.

Something snapped. Why had I thought about that fire? Was I being invited to reexamine my own petty sufferings, widowhood, unemployment, even the earache in the airplane, cold, robbery, the loss of personal treasures, the disappointment of going to Rome for a canonization never to reach the goal? Was this pilgrimage a metaphor for my own life outside religion? Was it a reminder that professional status and material things were valueless? Round and round these ideas turned. Angry to be disturbed, I was not converted and still I did not sleep.

In the morning, the sun shone, the world warmed and began to drip. We easily slid down out of the mountains past Gubbio and into Assisi, where more of Giotto's frescoes brought Saint Francis and Santa Clara into the canonical lessons. Woodward had explained how Saint Francis was right for his time with his youth, his message, his spirituality; his rapid canonization had rejuvenated the church. In a little shop on a street of Assisi, we found a soft gray-green sweater and skirt that I would wear to witness the elevation of a battered wife of Montreal to the ranks of Saint Francis—a saint for our time.

In Rome we shed the car, found our hotel, and went to the appointed rendezvous at the Collège Canadien near the Vatican. Père Constantin Bouchaud greeted us like long lost friends. He knew exactly where I fit in the story because he had shepherded the cause from his post in Rome. He introduced us to many sisters and priests who had already gathered. A special envelope held invitations to a celebration that evening at the residence of the Canadian ambassador to the Holy See and our tickets for the canonization the next day.

"Come with me," whispered Père Bouchaud and we followed him to an upstairs office where he proudly handed me a large book, bound in red cloth and lettered in gold, *Positio Super Miraculo*.[5]

The book contained documents about the miracle in the canonization process of Marguerite d'Youville. Inside were copies of Lise Normand's account, her records from the Ottawa General Hospital—information that I could not be shown all those years ago—, and the transcripts of our testimony at the ecclesiastical tribunal, with our initials scribbled on each page. The scientific articles that I had brought to the tribunal were also there, but the reproduction process had turned the careful pink highlighting into an impenetrable black, making the most important passages utterly illegible. It didn't matter, of course. The references were complete and a diligent researcher could easily find the rest. I could see this handsome book taking its place in the Vatican with thousands of other similar books from centuries of human experience, sources for that fancied medical history project on the nature of miracles.

"Thank you for showing me the book," I said.

"Take it," said Père Bouchaud, smiling and pushing the book back. "It's yours. We thought you would like to have a copy, being a historian and all." After the cold week of wandering and coping, the warmth of Canadian French, the joy of being recognized, and the promise of an adventure with new friends felt like home.

Back at the hotel I studied the big red book, which has become one of my most precious possessions. An introduction in Italian described the cast of characters: I had been misrepresented as a hematologist "di fama internazionale," but Jeanne later joked that it was only a typographic error—the passage had been meant to read "*in*fama nazionale." Eventually I found the discussion of "cure" versus "prolonged second remission." The committee had opted for "cure," but they did so with full recognition of the relapse and remission, coupled with a frank discussion of their usual implications, the possibility of "new" malignancies, and the difficulty of proclaiming cure in one still relatively young. We had done our bit; this canonization was squared with the canons of hematology.

In the late afternoon, we went sightseeing at the Roman Forum. Around its perimeters we noticed more saints: the jail that had held Saint Peter, a church to Saint Luke the physician apostle, and the basilica of Saints Cosmas and Damian. Like many early Christian churches, their basilica had been built in a former pagan temple. We had wanted to see the beautiful, sixth-century mosaic in the apse. But the location proved just as interesting. Nearby stood the three-column remains of the temple to another set of twins, Castor and Pollux, the Dioscuri (Figure 1.4). Between the temple and the Cosmas and Damian basilica lay the Fountain of Juturna, a well for ritual healing where archeologists had uncovered clay body parts left as votive offerings. Was there a connection between the early Christian twins and the ancient pagan twins? Were they all divine healers? Had the well served both religions as a site of healing? How could I find out?

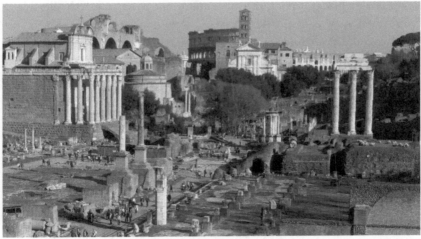

FIGURE 1.4 Roman forum with Basilica of Saints Cosmas and Damian, its rotunda and small cupola (middle distance, left center, to right of pillars), and three columns of Castor and Pollux temple (right), looking south with Coliseum in distance.

That night we joined a celebratory throng at the magnificent diplomatic residence of the Canadian ambassador to the Holy See near the ancient gate of Saint Sebastian. Some were ordinary citizens who had come from Varennes near Montreal to witness the elevation of their ancestor; most were clerics and nuns. We learned that back in Canada, a Montreal historian of Haïtian origin had just made a public protest over the canonization: he maintained that Mère d'Youville was an unworthy role model because she had kept slaves to help run her home and farms.[6] Could canonization be stayed at the last moment, like a launch of the space shuttle? What was his evidence? How could any sources remain that had not been studied? And above all, why had the professor waited so long to come forward with his information? The cause had been obvious for more than thirty years. Maybe he had been unable to draw attention to his concern until the media became involved. The news was disturbing, but it did not dampen the mood.

Everyone in the swirling, crowded rooms was drinking champagne. Kisses on both cheeks for old friends. One of the few other married couples, a man and woman from Oklahoma remotely descended from the family of the saint, told us how they had been following the cause for years. I was introduced to a familiar-looking woman. She was Marguerite Letourneau, the mother superior of the Grey Nuns who had sent me the invitation. She was also the sympathetic person who had noticed my pain on the descent into Rome a month-long week ago. In that atmosphere, coincidences were banal.

The following morning was cold and gray. As we walked across the Ponte Sant'Angelo in front of Hadrian's imposing tomb, a small band of adolescents walked menacingly toward us, too close, and grabbed my husband's coat. "No!" he said, drawing up his arms. They backed away, and we strode off with feeble dignity, probably too quickly to disguise our fear. Entering the huge embrace of Bernini's colonnade, we saw an enormous cloth banner of Marguerite d'Youville surrounded by children hanging from the west facade of Saint Peter's. The same image had been used in the cartoon biography and by the Exotik Travel Company. Was it naïve to be proud that a Canadian woman should be the focus of the Roman Catholic Church for an entire day?

A river of people flowed toward the basilica. At intervals, Swiss guards examined our coded tickets; some people were sent to the back of the nave. We moved closer and closer to the north transept where my husband was directed to a seat just behind the canopy and I was sent on to a pew in the second row in front of the altar. There beaming at me was Lise Normand, Dr. Drouin, Marguerite Letourneau, and a Sulpician father from Montreal. Beside us a troop of elegantly dressed Canadian diplomats eagerly took photographs of each other and of us. The superiority I felt over their sacrilegious popping of flash bulbs was considerably mollified by regret over our own stolen camera. Little did we know that back home in Canada, my family (and thousands of others) had risen early to watch and videotape the live television coverage. My mother and children had already spotted us on the screen and in his Toronto basement, my Polish-shtetl-born father-in-law was hooting with delight to see the balding head of his Jewish son just behind the chair of the Polish-born pontiff.

John Paul II arrived to a spontaneous burst of applause and the waving of the turquoise scarves, each with a daisy ("marguerite"), which we had been given at the entrance. I joined in enthusiastically, only later learning that this behavior was considered "gauche." Who knew? The pope bore a striking resemblance to my thesis advisor, Mirko Grmek, but he was smaller, stooped, and looked weary. I thought about his health problems and the scars of the 1981 assassination attempt that must hide under the layers of purple and white.

The order of service was printed in a richly illustrated booklet. Other saints were invoked, including those born in France who had died in Canada: Marguerite de Bourgeoys and the eight Jesuit martyrs of North America, including Jean de Brébeuf, Isaac Jogues, and the physician René Goupil. People who had experienced miracles were presented to the pope with offerings: Lise, radiant and strong; an elderly couple; and the little boy whose physician had refused to cooperate. A Grey Nun read a lesson in French, the life of Marguerite d'Youville was told, and an assistant made the formal plea that she be known as a saint. The pontiff replied in a single word, "Decernimus" (we determine it). Only God could "make" saints; humans merely "recognized" their sanctity. But they did so through rules—signs—guiding the interpretation of evidence that the soul was with God. Mass was celebrated in five languages, bells rang, the choir sang. And the service was over.

The sisters in my pew joined hands with Lise, Jeanne, and me, and led us behind a velvet curtain. I did not know where we were going and was anxious to find my husband again among the three thousand in the congregation. Suddenly I realized that we were at the end of a receiving line of perhaps twenty people, most Grey Nuns. The pope, who had already changed from his deep purple to a bright red cloak, was slowly coming toward us, guided by Père Bouchaud, shaking hands, receiving kisses on his ring, and bestowing blessings on the sisters, some of whom were moved to tears and fell on their knees. A tangle of black-clothed paparazzi with pointy shoes and slicked-back hair enveloped his every move in a hailstorm of popping lights.

Oh dear. "I wasn't expecting this," I said to Jeanne. "What do I do?"

"Well," she replied, "you're in Rome, do as . . ."

"I'm not going to kiss that ring, it can't be hygienic. Who knows where it's been?" My presence was an embodied insult, a fraud; anything I could do or say would only make it worse. In an instant Père Bouchaud was proudly introducing us as "the two doctors," attending physician and expert witness. John Paul II smiled and asked, "Are you members of the order?"

"Oh, no," we replied almost in unison, then the full implication of what he had asked dawned on me and I kept going so there should be no misunderstanding. "No, Holy Father," I said, "*Je suis une mère de famille!*"

Père Bouchaud did not miss a beat: "Just like the woman we have canonized to-day."

The pope's smile broadened and he looked back at us with an extra nod and blessing as he moved on to take Lise's hand. An official followed with a tray of little square packages that looked like After Eight mints but turned out to be rosaries like the one used by the pope.

"That was the pope! We met the pope! Jeanne, I had the pope on line! I blew it!" All those things I've been meaning to chat to him about: women priests, birth control, not to mention the lack of sources on his fifteenth-century predecessor, Innocent the VIII, who is supposed to have received the first blood transfusions by mouth. When would I ever get another opportunity? Instead, I had stood there trembling, grinning like an idiot, telling him that I was a mother. Would there be any pictures? In the excitement, I hadn't noticed the multiplicity of flashes that must have illuminated our ten-second audience, resulting in the many 8 x 10 color glossies that arrived in my office a few weeks later, a gift from clever Jeanne (Figure 1.5).

David found us there, gabbling about our experience.

"How was it for you?" we asked.

"Okay," he said. But he'd had some trouble understanding the little bells and the prayers of what turned out to be the ceremony of the mass. It would have been easy to explain beforehand, had we only realized.

"Have you never attended a mass before?"

"Well, why bother," he said, looking like his father, "if the pope is not officiating?"

We flew home the next day on reissued tickets. Back at the office, some pressing matters needed attention. Andréa, a senior student in medicine, was anxious to see me and had called several times. Within the hour, she burst

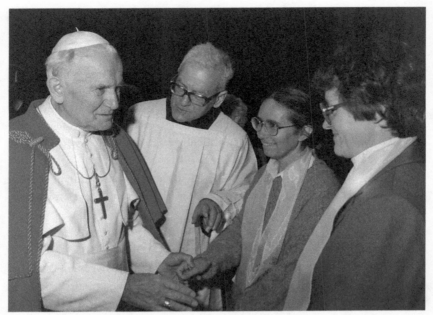

FIGURE 1.5 Pope John Paul II, Père Bouchaud, author, and Dr. Jeanne Drouin, December 9, 1990. Photo by Fotografia Felici, Rome.

into my office, apologizing for the rush. She wanted to do her final elective in medical history and the paperwork had to be signed that day, but she was worried I might not approve her project.

"No problem," I said. "Others have done history projects before."

"No, it's not the history," she explained, "it's the topic. I have a specific idea and I don't know what you'll think. It's sort of weird. I want to know more about Canada's first saint and the Grey Nuns' hospitals, but I couldn't discuss it with you because you weren't here."

She must be joking. "Andréa, you know where I was, don't you?"

"No, but you've been gone just over a week, and with term just ending! And you probably don't even know what I'm talking about because you won't have seen the papers."

I told her where I had been. She turned pale; I think I did too, and maybe a little bell started ringing far away.

"Then you won't mind," she said softly.

I picked up the phone and called Marguerite Letourneau in Montreal. "I have here a medical student who would like to know more about Saint Marie-Marguerite d'Youville. Could she come to study in your archives?" I sensed that the mother superior was smiling: "That is precisely what we wanted. The young doctor is more than welcome."

Throughout this adventure, I kept thinking that miracles grew harder and harder to come by in this age of technology, skepticism, and speed. Surely, the church was vexed by the relative subordination of theology in the decision-making process to a committee of medical professionals whose years of training and whose very language were constructed to reduce human experience to molecules and probabilities. Now, I was far less certain.

Lise Normand continues in miraculously good health more than twenty years after our journey to Rome. Had she been healed of fever and bruising two hundred years ago, no one would have seen a miracle. Two centuries ago, leukemia had not yet been recognized; the medical rules to identify this disease, based on microscopic study of the blood, had not been developed; nor had its dismal survival rates been defined.

We tend to think of diseases as autonomous beings, but historians know that diseases are only ideas, metaphysical entities. In a sense, they are merely theories about illness, which tend to favor objective, passive explanations at the expense of the subjective and active stories of people. Without the nineteenth-century "invention" of leukemia and its sinister prognosis, there would be no miraculous cures of that disease today. In fact, microscopes, blood smears, and special stains do not reduce but rather open up a whole new realm of possibility for miracles, which have been and continue to be conditioned by science. A miracle is something that exceeds our expectations, that defies the "rules"— be they scientific or spiritual—that we humans construct to explain, identify, label, and comprehend our natural experience. So my own definition of "miracle" is simple: it is a thing of wonder, a transcendent experience, inexplicable by current human wisdom.

As for disease, so it is for saints. Humans have invented rules to order experience and facilitate comprehension—in diagnosing disease and in detecting sanctity. But unlike their medical counterparts, the rules of canonization accommodate and rely on the *subjective* account. Could a miracle have been perceived in her healing, if Lise herself did not attribute it to the saint? Canonization does not "create" a saint so much as it allows the faithful to recognize that events, which have been ascribed to the intercession of the spirit, cannot be explained in any other way, including the best of contemporary science. These rules create confidence in the attribution of divine intervention.

ON THAT LENGTHY journey to Saint Peter's Basilica, I may not have been converted to formal religion, but I was brought to acknowledge two truths that I had previously managed to avoid—truths that ran against all my medical training.

First, miracles exist. They simply fall outside the honestly made and well-established boundaries of what two radically different sets of human rules—medicine and religion—teach us to expect. Since there is no limit to the diversity of our existence, miracles can happen every day, and, on some level, science makes them possible. That was a big revelation.

Second, saints participate in the suffering and hopes of people in our world. They may not have been important to me as a skeptical physician—but it was unrealistic to ignore their importance in the lives of my patients. I began to see saints everywhere and, disconcertingly, they all seemed to be dabbling in medicine whether they had once been doctors or not.

2

Doctor Twins

FROM CYRRHUS TO TORONTO

The flood of the sick at the Saints Cosmas and Damian shrine was not some relic of paganism; rather it arose from an essential impulse of the human spirit, in all times and all beliefs, the impulse leads to Healers, whatever name they bear... all possible healers have responded to these two constant facts: human misery and unshakeable confidence in divine Beneficence.
—FESTUGIÈRE, *Sainte Thecle, Saints Côme et Damien, 1971, 94–95.*[1]

JUST A FEW months after the canonization, I was walking in Toronto's Little Italy when a poster stapled to a telephone pole brought me up short (Figure 2.1). It announced the feast-day celebration of the doctor saints, Cosmas and Damian, those twin martyrs whose ancient basilica stands in the Roman Forum.

The neighborhood—south of College Street, north of Dundas Street, and extending west of Bathurst Street for several blocks—was, and still is, very Italian. Scholarly studies document its history and sociology.[2] During my medical school days in the early 1970s, I lived there in a second-floor flat with a rickety balcony and a shared bathroom. The narrow, Victorian-gothic houses were painted bright colors, each brick outlined by contrasting lines on the mortar. They boasted tiny, well-kept gardens with wrought iron fences and ornate statues, often Virgin-in-the-half-shell variety. On summer evenings, families gathered on the porches talking across lawns and laneways; sometimes they sang. The Mediterranean grocery across the street sold delicious, salty bread and wrinkled, black olives from a murky barrel. My landlady, Silvana, was younger than I, but already she had three children and always wore black. Early in the morning, I could hear her footsteps and those of women like her, young and old, all dressed in mourning, walking to mass at Saint Francis of Assisi Church on nearby Grace Street.

CITTA' DI TORONTO
FESTEGGIAMENTI IN ONORE DEI SANTI MEDICI

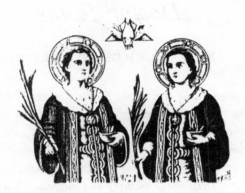

S. COSMA E DAMIANO
DOMENICA, 27 SETTEMBRE, 1992. PRESSO LA CHIESA DI:
SAN FRANCESCO D'ASSISI
GRACE ST. E MANSFIELD AVE. (ZONA PICCOLA ITALY)

S. COSMA E DAMIANO: CONTINUANO A VIVERE ATTRAVERSO I SECOLI CON LA LORO IMMAGINE IN QUEI MOLTISSIMI E MOLTISSIMI MEDICI, E' HANNO TRASMESSO COME SACRA EREDITA' L'ESEMPIO DI UN GENEROSO DISINTERESSE. L'AMORE VERSO CRISTO SOTTO LE SPOGLIE DEL MALATO, SPECIE SE POVERO, IL SENSO DELLA PIU' ADORABILE MODESTIA, SIGILLO INCONFONDIBILE DELLA VERA GRANDEZZA, COSI' LA FESTA DI S. COSMA E DAMIANO SI RINNOVERA' OGNI GIORNO NELLA NOSTRA VITA, PREGATE PER NOI!

PROGRAMMA RELIGIOSO

SERA DEL 24, 25, 26 SETTEMBRE ALLE ORE 7:00 P.M.
TRIDICO IN PREPARAZIONE DELLA FESTA
CON P. ANTONIO NARDOIANNI, O.F.M.

DOMENICA MATTINA: S. MESSA IN CHIESA
ORE 8:00 & 10:15 A.M., IN ITALIANO
ORE 9:00 & 11:30 A.M., IN INGLESE

ALLE ORE 2:00 P.M., MESSA SOLENNE IN CHIESA CON P. ANTONIO NARDOIANNI, O.F.M.
ALLE ORE 3:00 P.M., PROCESSIONE PER LE VIE DELLA PARROCCHIA, E'
LA VENERAZIONE DELLA RELIQUIA

ALLE ORE 4:00 P.M. SPETTACOLO MUSICALE CON ...
"CITY LIGHTS" - IVAN SANTILLI

| Bazaar | Pizza | Porchetta | Sausages |
| Games | Popcorn | Candy Floss | Pasta e Cece |

FIGURE 2.1 Poster for Toronto feast, 1992.

The poster on the telephone pole came from that same Saint Francis church. But I could not recall a feast for the medical saints when I had lived in Little Italy two decades earlier. Was it new? Or had I simply failed to notice it? Where did it come from, and why? It never occurred to me that finding the answers to those questions would take twenty years and fill the pages of a book.

Who Are the Doctor Saints?

The Internet had yet to be invented. I started with encyclopedias and soon found that many people had written about these saints. Physicians Cosmas and Damian were twin brothers martyred for their Christian faith in the violent persecutions waged by the Roman Emperor Diocletian, who reigned between 283 and 303 AD. Evidence pertaining to their lives is vague and problematic, stemming mostly from legends and archival fragments, deemed "entirely uncertain and unknown."[3] Four manuscripts in the Vatican archives were summarized by Stiltingo for the *Acta Sanctorum*, which is the authoritative compendium of saints prepared by the Bollandist fathers in Belgium. Cosmas and Damian are said to have been born in the mid-third century at Aegae in the Roman province of Cicilia (now Çukurova, Turkey) on the Bay of Alexandretta (Iskenderun), within the northeastern corner of the Mediterranean. The name of the saints' birthplace may have commemorated another Aegae, the original capital of Macedonia. Their alleged birthplace is now identified as the small town of Ayas in the Yumurtalik district of Turkey's Adana province.

Most sources suggest that Cosmas and Damian were neither Greek nor Roman, but of "eastern" descent; some call them "oriental," others "Arabs." They studied medicine in what is now Syria. Refusing payment for their work, they came to be known as the "Anargyroi," a Greek word signifying "without silver"—those who take no money. The generous brothers performed wonderful cures of ailments such as blindness, paralysis, and fever; they raised the dead and expelled a breast serpent, and while doing so they proselytized their religion. Willing to offer help wherever it was needed, the brothers also healed a sick camel. Once, a woman by the name of Palladia insisted that Damian accept three eggs as a token of gratitude for her cure (Figure 2.2). Not wishing to offend, Damian accepted the eggs, but his lapse angered Cosmas, who declared that he would not be buried with his twin. The bitter conflict was resolved through the intercession of yet another camel, one who could talk. Their deeds were described by the seventh-century

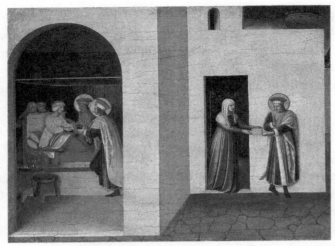

FIGURE 2.2 Fra Angelico, The Healing of Palladia. National Gallery of Art, Washington, DC.

Sophronius of Jerusalem, and in early manuscripts, the thirteenth-century *Golden Legend* as well as the *Acta Sanctorum*.[4]

During the persecutions of Diocletian, Cosmas and Damian together with their three brothers, Anthimus, Leontius, and Euprepius, were tried by Lysias, governor of Cilicia. The gruesome torture and killing is an oft-repeated story that inspired many paintings, including numerous works by Fra Angelico. They were thrown in the sea, but angels retrieved them; they were set alight at the stake, but the flames did not consume them; they were shot by archers, but the arrows turned back on the assailants; they were stoned and crucified, for hours, without effect. Finally they were beheaded (Figures 2.3 and 2.4). If this hyper-resistant vitality was connected to their healing occupation, we are not told. Reports differ, but the Bollandists situate their death in the year AD 297.

The remains of Cosmas and Damian were carried inland and east to the town of Cyr or Cyrrhus, now a ruin and extensive archeological site called al-Nabi Houri in Syria.[5] Founded as a Hellenistic colony and already five hundred years old, Cyrrhus had converted to Christianity many years earlier; a basilica was either expanded or newly erected over the twins' tomb. Other saints were also buried there, making the town a site of pilgrimage, also known as Hagiopolis.

Cosmas and Damian became prominent martyrs at a key moment, just before freedom and power were extended to the faith. The persecutions

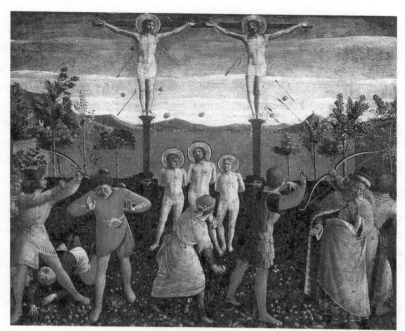

FIGURE 2.3 Fra Angelico, Cosmas and Damian and their brothers crucified, stoned, and shot with arrows. Alte Pinakothek, Munich.

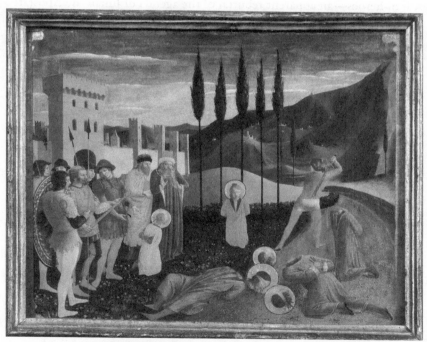

FIGURE 2.4 Fra Angelico, Altarpiece of St. Mark: The Decapitation of Cosmas and Damian and their brothers. Louvre, Paris, France. Photo Credit: Scala/Art Resource, NY.

ended with the abdication of Diocletian, and religious freedom was promised in the Edict of Milan in AD 313. Constantine proclaimed Christianity as the state religion in AD 324. Soon after, a bishop of Cyr attended the important Council of Nicea in 325. In the mid-fourth century, however, the pagan emperor Julian, called the Apostate, attempted to de-Christianize the empire. He discredited the practice of venerating martyrs as a throwback to the hero-worship of the ancient religion, which he admired. He also revived the cult of Asklepios (Aesculapius in Latin), the pagan god of medicine, in opposition to that of Jesus.[6] But his efforts failed. Julian was the last non-Christian emperor. His death around AD 363 unleashed a vigorous celebration of saints, especially of the recent martyrs who had suffered and died for their religion.

In the following century, Theodoret (d. before 466), one of the early church fathers, became bishop of Cyrrhus. He restored a number of the Roman works at the site, including aqueducts, bridges, and baths. Seemingly familiar with medicine, he was intrigued by its parallels with theology. His metaphorical treatise, entitled "Treatment of Hellenistic Diseases," includes an apology for the worship of martyrs in opposition to the pagan cult of heroes—an apparent rebuttal of the agenda of Julian the Apostate.[7] Pilgrims were said to have come to Cyrrhus in large numbers to venerate Cosmas and Damian, although Theodoret's extant writings do not mention the saints.

Cyrrhus had a stormy history. Twice occupied by Persians prior to Theodoret, it was finally captured by Arab armies in 637. Stones from its basilica were said to have been carried to Aleppo, forty-five miles away, for use in construction of the great Umayyad Mosque. Begun in the eighth century, this enormous mosque covered the sites of an earlier Roman temple and a Christian basilica that had featured a fifth-century chapel to the medical saints.[8]

Back in Cyrrhus, the Roman bridges and an early third-century hexagonal mausoleum remain, but nothing now designates the burial site of the Christian twins. Their graves may have vanished. Nevertheless, within a century of their deaths, Cosmas and Damian were venerated in Jerusalem and throughout the Roman Empire, and their wondrous healings continued. Many were cures effected in dreams while patients slept in their sanctuaries, a process strikingly similar to the "incubation" practices of ancient temple medicine.

In the prevalent rite of incubation, people who were sick would visit a complex that included doctors, priests, baths, temples, and a hostel, if not a hospital. After suitable preparation, both physical and spiritual, they would make offerings and sleep in the temple, hoping for dreams that might entail a visit or a message from the god. It was a lifestyle form of cure, not too different from health retreats or spas in our own time. Because sources on incubation are so numerous, the deep connection between temple medicine and Christian practices was recognized more than a hundred years ago.[9]

A celebrity miracle served to enhance the reputation of the medical saints in the Byzantine Empire. The emperor Justinian, who reigned from 527 to 565, attributed his recovery from an illness to their intercession. In gratitude, he restored the town of Cyrrhus and dedicated two more churches to Cosmas and Damian in Constantinople, bringing the late sixth-century total in that city to four, one of which adjoined a hospital and was called the "Kosmidion."[10] Greek manuscripts present forty-eight miracles said to have been worked by Cosmas and Damian in one of these churches; the supplicants included pagans, Christians, and Jews.[11] The stories are sufficiently detailed to allow a modest reconstruction of the church emphasizing its connection to the hospital.[12] Most are healings from disease: swellings, paralysis, blindness, deafness, fractures, tumors, sores, abscesses, and problems of the sexual organs; at least one entailed incubation. A few provide unusual twists: in anger over his dismissal, the monastery's cattle herder plans to set fire to the buildings; two men appear in a fog and expose his secret, leading him to repent. Another man who wrongly suspects his wife of infidelity is stricken with an eye disease; the saints promise a cure but only with the application of breast milk from a pure woman. The wife's milk proves her virtue, saving the man's sight and his marriage.[13]

The saints' most famous cure is the "miracle of the black leg" (Figure 2.5). A white man with a festering, possibly gangrenous leg slept in their basilica in the healing ritual of incubation. The saints replaced his sick leg with that of a dead black man ("Aethiop") recently interred in the local cemetery. Some versions describe this miracle as one worked during the saints' lives; others claim it was posthumous and took place in the Roman basilica. Portrayed numerous times by artists, the miracle of the black leg and its multiple renditions in images and words have attracted scholars of art, history, literature, and semiotics.[14] It is used often for medical purposes, and surgical journals are fond of citing the Anargyroi as patrons of organ transplantation.[15] This proclivity led one exasperated historian to wonder "why intelligent and educated people, such as transplant surgeons, engage in producing a sort of history that for many historians looks little short of absurd."[16]

In early Christianity, the blending of medicine and religion was entrenched in symbols and practice: sick people routinely sought help at monasteries and

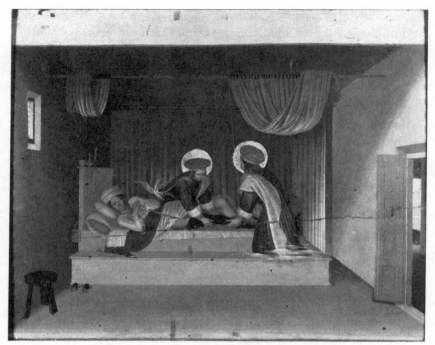

FIGURE 2.5 Fra Angelico, Altarpiece of Saint Mark: Predella with the Deacon Justinian being healed by Saints Cosmas and Damian [miracle of the black leg]. Museo di S. Marco, Florence, Italy. Photo Credit: Scala/Art Resource.

churches where wise monks offered both prayers and medicines. These centers usually included a *xenodochion*, or hospice for strangers, a facility that blended care with accommodation.[17] Incubation continued there. The altar cloths of the Hagia Sofia are said to have been decorated with images of hospitals.[18] At Sykeon in Galatie in the center of present-day Turkey, the charismatic sixth-century healer Theodore hung an icon of the twin saints above his bed and attributed his own recovery from illness to their intercession.[19]

Shrines to Cosmas and Damian were established in many other places. Their first church in "the west" was said to be founded in Subiaco by Saint Benedict (480–542), and the Benedictine monks maintained a long tradition of veneration.[20] Ravenna and Athens also practiced early devotion to the twin doctors. The original building of their basilica in the Roman Forum had once been the library of the Temple of Peace (also called the forum of Vespasian), dating to about AD 75 and is said to have been constructed to celebrate the conquest of Jerusalem (Figures 1.4 and 2.6). On an outer wall, the great map of Rome, the Forma Urbis, was suspended in the year AD 211.[21] In the early sixth century, Pope Felix IV, who served from AD 526 to 530, had it converted into a Christian basilica to honor the twin doctors. The original entrance was from the forum through a round vestibule that had been erected as a shrine to Jupiter Stator; later, the noble Maxentius dedicated it in honor of his dead son, Romulus, deified in AD 307. The apse of the basilica was decorated with a brilliant mosaic, the one that we had seen in December 1990. It depicts Christ flanked on either side by the doctor saints with Saints Peter and Paul. It is said to be one of the earliest mosaics to display Jesus in a Semitic fashion. Lambs file around the bottom margin to represent the apostles, a blue band signifies the River Jordan, and a pink flamingo on a palm tree represents the Holy Spirit.

From at least the fourth century and probably earlier, Christians venerated relics of saints. Donation or theft of martyrs' bodily remains served to link far-flung churches in a newly emerging tradition.[22] In 592, prior to the dismantling of the Cyrrhus basilica, Pope Gregory the Great is said to have brought some or all of the saints' bones from Syria to the Roman basilica, where he placed them under the altar.[23] From Rome, small relics were transported widely—parts of a skull, a fragment of an arm, a finger, a rib.

According to an eleventh-century historian, the Bremen archbishop Adaldag brought the skulls from Rome around the year 965. They were then allegedly rediscovered in the cathedral choir by his successor, Burchard Grelle, in 1335.[24] Around 1420, a magnificent oak reliquary with gold and silver covering was made to shelter and display them. In 1649 the relics were sold by the newly Protestant Bremen and then translated to Saint Michael's Church of Munich, where they are still encased in the ornate reliquary. Earlier, many of the remaining bones were plundered from Rome in the late twelfth century by the French seigneur Jean de Beaumont (also Bellemont), who was returning from a crusade; he placed them in Paris and Luzarches.[25] The skulls of Cosmas and Damian were also said to have been given in 1581 to Las Descalzas Reales, a Poor Clares Franciscan convent in Madrid; these crania were inspected in 1935 by an anthropologist who concluded that they were ancient and had belonged to men who died in their fifties.[26] Vienna also has a pair of skulls preserved in a neo-Gothic reliquary in the Valentinskapelle of Saint Stephen's Cathedral. Even Stiltingo, the eighteenth-century author of the entry in the *Acta Sanctorum*, expressed doubt that all these relics could belong to the twin healers; he suggested that they may have been mixed with those of their three brothers.[27] The list of sites where their bones reside suggests a mass of organic material far greater than that which would normally comprise two human skeletons.

Whether or not the saints had ever existed, by the eleventh century, people all over Europe believed that they had. With or without relics, numerous shrines, towns, monasteries, and churches were dedicated to their honor all over the continent. By 675, Toledo had a monastery under their protection; Cordoba had another in the ninth century. In France, the fifth-century Saint Germain promoted their cult. The Saint Côme priory on an island in the Loire at Tours traces its origin to the late eleventh century; five hundred years later the poet Pierre de Ronsard lived and died there. In France more than a hundred places now venerate the saints, many, but not all, prompted by a gift of relics.[28] Anneliese Wittmann identified thirty-eight sites with objects of devotion in Switzerland, forty-one in Austria, thirty-three in the low countries, and nearly three hundred in Germany.[29]

In Italy, the passing of each epidemic would leave a cluster of chapels and shrines to honor the santi medici, almost, said one writer, "as if they were vo-tives of thanksgiving."[30] That country boasts more than 180 sites dedicated to the saints, while Rome had no fewer than eight churches.[31] Of these, only two remain: the basilica in the Roman Forum and San Cosimato in Trastevere. Founded in the mid-tenth century and consecrated in 1066 by Pope Alexander II, San Cosimato included a *xenodochion* as well as a convent, in the arrangement typical of early churches. Its history and daily life were documented by a sixteenth-century nun, Orsola Fromicini, who was the daughter of a doctor.[32] In her time, the monastery contained two cloisters, a garden, and vineyards. Gradually, its main function became a hospital, and in 1892 most of the old monastery was demolished to make way for the new Ospedale Nuovo della Regina Margherita.[33] A fading fresco of Saint Cosmas adorns a wall in the present-day pharmacy.

Other churches and shrines are found in the Czech Republic, Portugal, and Spain. One of the most beautiful depictions of the saints' lives is the fifteenth-century retable above the altar of their chapel in the cathedral of Barcelona.[34] Their statues are prominent on the Charles Bridge in Prague. Inheriting the Byzantine tradition, Eastern Europe, Asia, North Africa, and the Middle East also have sites dedicated to their memory, in countries such as Croatia, Poland, Slovenia, Bulgaria, Egypt, Syria, and the Ukraine.[35] No fewer than three pairs of twins, all named Cosmas and Damian, were venerated in the Eastern Orthodox religion, each with separate feast days, but all are thought to have originated as variations upon the same theme.[36]

Following European colonization, Mexico, Brazil, Paraguay, Argentina, the United States, and Canada also had churches, convents, and towns under the protection of the saints. It seems that the twin healers arrived in the Americas around the same time as the first European physicians. The church that claims to be the oldest in Brazil was founded under their patronage at Igarassu in 1535. On the saints' feast day in September, Brazilian children are given candy.

Back in Rome, structural and decorative changes to the forum basilica became necessary in the sixteenth century. Rubble and silt had accumulated in the forum through centuries of neglect; it meant that visitors were obliged to descend a staircase to reach the basilica floor at the original level of the forum. Owing to long-standing blockage of the cloaca maxima—the sewer that drained the originally swampy area of the forum—the basilica floor was often damp, the stench unbearable, and the air insalubrious. The raising of the floor began in 1626, bringing it to the higher street level and improving the atmosphere. These renovations cut the church in half horizontally; they also created new side chapels and a painted, coffered ceiling, thereby mutilating some of the mosaics. New decorations and frescoes were added. The elevated floor effectively lowered the ceiling and brought the congregation closer to the great mosaic in the apse, which now appears as much behind the altar as above it.[37]

Secular and professional institutions of physicians, pharmacists, and surgeons also venerated the saints across Europe. The Confrérie (later Collège) Saint Côme in Paris was founded to serve surgeons in 1260; it later enjoyed the patronage of Louis XIII, who had been born on the saints' feast in 1601. In the late seventeenth century, the Collège constructed an elegant, round amphitheater for anatomical instruction; the building still stands in the rue de l'Ecole de Médecine off the Boulevard Saint Michel near les Cordeliers.[38] From the fifteenth century, the pharmacists of Rome fixed the locus of activity of their "Nobile Collegio Chimico Farmaceutico" in San Lorenzo in Miranda, the church next door to the forum basilica of Cosmas and Damian. It, too, was a revamped pagan temple, originally dedicated to Faustina and Antoninus; the six mighty columns across its façade remain notwithstanding the major renovations in the early seventeenth century (Figure 2.6). Even in earlier times and other places, pharmacists had designated Saint Damian as another patron. As a result, Damian is often identified in images as the pharmacist saint who holds pots of medicine or plants, while Cosmas is the surgeon or physician who holds a book or another instrument of the trade.[39]

In addition to the traditional hagiographies that recite the lives and wonders of these saints, several scholars have conducted sophisticated

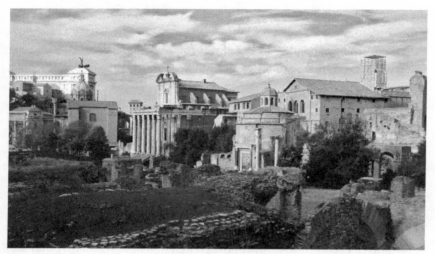

FIGURE 2.6 Basilica of Saints Cosmas and Damian with its rotunda and San Lorenzo in Miranda with its columns to the left, looking north east.

investigations of their cult. In particular, Marie-Louise David-Danel analyzed their iconography, providing an extensive repertoire of sites and artifacts throughout Europe. She observed that the various portrayals of the doctor brothers reflect the historical development of medicine itself.[40] With the palm branch of martyrs, they sometimes hold books, spatulae, pots of ointment, mortars and pestles, urinals, scalpels, blood-letting instruments, thermometers, and even test tubes. Altarpieces and other devotional works crafted for the Medici family of Florence meant that their patrons, the santi medici, were often depicted by the hands of brilliant artists: Fra Angelico, Sano di Pietro, Bicci di Lorenzo, Fra Filippo Lippi, Taddeo Gaddi, Sandro Botticelli, and other great names of the Renaissance.[41] Some artists deliberately placed Medici family faces on the robed bodies of the doctor saints.[42] A host of guidebooks and spiritual publications feature local festivals, usually opening with a short biography of the holy twins, some of which have been written with careful attention to scholarly sources.[43] Others are transcriptions of manuscripts in Greek concerning their lives and miracles.[44]

Wittmann charted the growth and decline of their popular devotion with special attention to shrines in Sicily and Germany, showing how their veneration had been eclipsed by the rise of a local saint.[45] Between 1970 and 1993, the late Pierre Julien of Paris extended this research by meticulously collating and examining sites of feast-day celebrations and by drawing attention to their iconography, especially within the history of pharmacy.

Sensitive to the fascination of popular devotion, he assembled an enormous personal collection of prints and objects pertaining to the santi medici in both low and high art, and he published articles using the artifacts as his primary sources. In these objects, twinliness seems as significant as the medical attributes.

The saints' feast was set in the *Calendarium Romanum* as September 27, but it was changed to September 26 in 1969 to avoid a conflict with the feast of St. Vincent de Paul, a post-Congregation saint who also was associated with healing and whose existence is not in dispute. The Roman basilica adopted the change, but many places adhere to September 27. Until the Second Vatican Council in 1962, Cosmas and Damian were named in the liturgy. As a result, older Catholics recognized them readily when I described my interest; younger ones looked at me blankly.

Ancient Twins and the Genealogical Theory

I was keen to discover how the saints might relate to Castor and Pollux, divine twins of a distant, pagan past. This possibility had suggested itself by the proximity of the basilica to the temple, and the Juturna fountain lying between them. The literature on Cosmas and Damian was vast, erudite, and eclectic, and as Pierre Julien observed, the precise reasons for the apparition and extension of the cult "escape us still."[46] Sifting slowly through the voluminous material, I was slightly disappointed, though not surprised, to learn that I had been scooped. The possible connection to earlier twin deities had already been spotted, and more than a century before. But here the sources diverged widely into partisan perspectives; some argued that the connections were obvious; others were strongly opposed to the recognition of such links.

Those who perceived firm connections to the past contend that similar parallels exist throughout the religion—for example, between Artemis (or Diana) in Ephesus and the Virgin Mary as well as between the healing god Asklepios (Aesculapius) and Jesus or the medical saints.[47] For them, the cult of pagan heroes relates directly to that of Christian saints through a kind of "syncretism." Consequently, the medical saints would have resonated with converts accustomed to the veneration of other twins, such as Castor and Pollux (Kastor and Polydeukes in Greek), also known as the Dioscuri. These are the twin heroes remembered in the constellation Gemini.[48] Several clerics readily described these parallels to me, untroubled by the implications.[49]

According to the myth, the Dioscuri were born to Leda, the beautiful wife of a king who had been seduced by the god Zeus disguised as a swan. The twins had been particularly dear to ancient Romans for appearing as horsemen and heralding a decisive military victory around the year 495 BC at Lake Regillus, which is now a dry volcanic crater southeast of Rome. The temple to Castor and Pollux in the Roman Forum was built to honor this victory; its three standing columns are a familiar sight. Gigantic statues to the Dioscuri occupy prominent positions in Rome. Though naked, they and their horses still fight the battle of Lake Regillus in the piazza outside the Quirinale Palace, and they stand guard atop the staircase leading to Michelangelo's elegant Campidoglio on Capitoline Hill. Sailors also looked to the divine twins for protection from storms.[50]

Further supporting the links to antiquity, one of the many miracles ascribed to Cosmas and Damian was connected to the Dioscuri, although the Roman version of the pagan pair were not particularly known for healing works. A man was sent by other pagans to the basilica having been told it was for Castor and Pollux; he was healed after repudiating their names "with horror."[51] Two other miracles have Cosmas and Damian saving a lad from drowning and guiding his ship to safety, just as the Dioscuri were wont to do.[52]

Scholars also point to evidence from the early church fathers who recognized how the pagan practice of hero worship could be related to the Christian veneration of martyr saints.[53] In some places, people honored deities from both religions at once. Another pair of third-century martyrs, Cyrus and John, one a doctor, were venerated at a shrine near Alexandria that was also sacred to Isis, whose devotion endured for at least two hundred more years.[54] Patriarch of Constantinople and a hospital founder, John Chrysostom (ca 347–407), wrote that some early Christian peoples still worshipped Castor and Pollux.[55]

Among scholars inclined to accept pre-Christian influences, some speculate on the possibility that both the pagan and the Christian twins were descended from an even older but more obscure set of twins venerated in the prototypical religion of the Indo-European peoples. Oral traditions from generation to generation have been invoked to explain other "astonishing coincidences" in the creation myths of India and Europe.[56] Evidence for this hypothesis with respect to Cosmas and Damian stems from the fact that twins with healing powers were also known in the Hindu pantheon.[57] Their name, Nasatyas or Asvins, has been linked to the stem of the German verb meaning to convalesce or recover: "genesen."[58] The late-first-century historian Tacitus claimed that the peoples of Germania venerated the Alci, twin deities whom the Romans interpreted as Castor and Pollux.[59] Norse and

Baltic traditions also recognized pairs of heroic siblings.[60] According to the interpretation of the apocryphal Acts of Thomas, Jesus's mortal twin was Thomas; the name in Syriac means "twin," as does "Didymus," the name given to Thomas in Greek.[61] This story too has been construed as a sign of the existence of an earlier cult of twins.

Based on these views, Cosmas and Damian could be descended from a long, unbroken line of divine twins that has traversed several millennia and religions. Intriguing as these suggestions may be, efforts to actually connect the saints to other twin gods are fraught with contradictions and lacunae.

Conversely, some Christian writers oppose the links with pagan antiquity and other religions. For them, saints Cosmas and Damian were real people who served God and died for their faith. Attempts to trace their origins in a non-Christian past might be intellectually attractive, but the parallels are construed as mere coincidence. Portraying them as derivatives of a more distant time must be defeated with solid evidence and logical argument. Thus the erudite Delehaye admitted to survivals of ancient practices, but he attacked those "obstinately bent on finding examples of suspect custom everywhere" and accused a proponent of the pagan links of having a "veritable obsession with the Dioscuri." He pointed out that the church "has never ceased to fight against [the links], varying her tactics with different degrees of success."[62]

Some go so far as to dismiss the efforts to unravel the connections with antiquity as a waste of time. Instead, they accept the stories of the saints literally, as history, or they adopt a detachment that stems more from anthropology than faith. Without denying parallels and similarities, Peter R. L. Brown insisted on the important differences between pagan and Christian attitudes to the dead.[63] Festugière, cited in the epigraph to this chapter, claimed that proving that souvenirs of paganism may have existed in the Kosmidion is far less important than noticing the "essential impulse of the human spirit" that will identify healers "whatever name they bear." The persistence of Cosmas and Damian, he continued, is "not that they succeeded Castor and Pollux, but that Asklepios, the Dioscuri, the medical saints, and all the healers possible respond to two constant facts: human misery and unshakeable confidence in divine Beneficence."[64]

Other complexities can be found in this debate. Some Christian believers recognize the existence of saintly people, but they invoke a "degradation narrative" that looks on the veneration of saints and their relics as a kind of magical corruption infesting the purity of the early church.[65] Holy people were assigned new and more desirable attributes: for example, in early texts, Jesus was described as a "healer" of both bodies and souls, but a "dramatic explosion" of physical healings occurred in the late fourth century.[66] These believers contend that after the persecutions ended, the religion became popular with so-called "nominal Christians," who retained their pagan traditions, as opposed to the more devout early Christians, who had severed connections with their past, welcomed illness as a good, and were ready to be eaten by lions.[67] Some went so far as to suggest that the expanding church deliberately promoted devotion to empty homologous figures simply to make the new religion seem comprehensible, familiar, and palatable, thereby enhancing its appeal to pagans.[68] Others maintain that the syncretism resulting from a perceived "democratization" of early Christianity could be a fabrication of scholarship.[69]

I was getting confused. The sources participated in the interpretation, championing one view over another and obscuring the social function of all healing cults. As with any historical endeavor, writer bias colors not only the analysis, but also the selection of evidence. In the case of the medical saints, authors seem to be either absolute believers or absolute skeptics with little middle ground.[70]

Did Cosmas and Damian originate in protohistory? The answer was a definite "maybe." But these erudite studies had focused mostly on Europe. And none could explain what the medical saints were doing in Toronto on that September day in 1991.

Cosmas and Damian in Toronto

I could not go to Toronto for that feast day, so I appealed to my best friend, Anita Johnston. We had been at medical school together, living for two years in the late 1960s in the same nurses' residence because there had been no residence for women medical students. A year ahead of me, this fearless redhead had been a major factor in my survival with her patience, experience, and earthy sense of humor. After two years, we saved our friendship by *not* living together, and that is when I found my apartment in Little Italy. Having trained as a psychiatrist and psychoanalyst, Anita was now living in one of those narrow Victorian-gothic houses on Grace Street, which was why I had happened upon the poster in the first place. Armed with her camera (paper photographs or slides in those days), she shot a whole roll of film to document the well-attended mass and procession with statues of the saints, a band, special banners, and robes.

She described the event on the phone: "The police stopped traffic on both College and Dundas; the parade was very Italian—maybe even Sicilian, with a band and singing." She was sure that she heard a tarantella. No question, this was big—so big that it must be new since our student days. Or had we simply been blinkered to the religion all around us in our student pursuit of what we thought was a science?

I called the church and was referred to the former parish priest, Father Raffaele (Ralph) Paonessa, who had since been transferred to a church in another neighborhood. He explained that lively festivals are a feature of the yearly cycle of this parish. At Christmas, a life-sized, illuminated crèche occupies the outer wall of the church and carols are played on a loudspeaker. At Easter, a passion play receives media attention. Celebration of the feast of Cosmas and Damian blended well with these other seasonal practices. In answer to my question, Father Paonessa speculated hesitantly that the Toronto parish may have been the first city in Canada to celebrate the santi medici; however, he readily cited other healing shrines in our country, such as Sainte Anne-de-Beaupré, the Oratoire Saint Joseph, and the Jesuit Martyrs shrine. But this tradition did not originate with the gothic gray stone building itself. It came much later. The parish was established in 1903, originally for Irish Catholics, and the church was designed in 1910 by architect A. W. Holmes, who had also designed Saint Michael's College at the University of Toronto. The church became Italianized gradually between 1957, when the nearby St. Agnes parish changed from serving Italian immigrants to Portuguese ones.[71] Father Ralph confirmed that the celebration did not exist when I had lived in Little Italy. It began in 1987.

The events follow a regular pattern that Anita had observed and Father Paonessa confirmed (Figure 2.7). On September 27, or the nearest Sunday to it, a special mass is said in the large church; the life-sized, solid-wood, polychrome statues of Cosmas and Damian mounted on a common base are moved from their usual position, near the west door, to a prominent place near the front. They are decorated with flowers and long ribbons of money, mostly twenty-dollar bills joined by dressmaker pins, although a few fifty- and one-hundred-dollar denominations are apparent too. At the end of the mass, the heavy statues are carried down the aisle, out the main door, down the staircase, to a rolling dais waiting below. The congregation follows and mills about on the steps and in the street. Outside, the band plays music, both solemn and jolly, including marches and tarantellas. A procession forms led by the priests. The statues are borne along by men pushing the rolling dais, a few groups carrying banners follow, and behind them walk people who are profoundly religious, some who are sick, and some who have sick friends

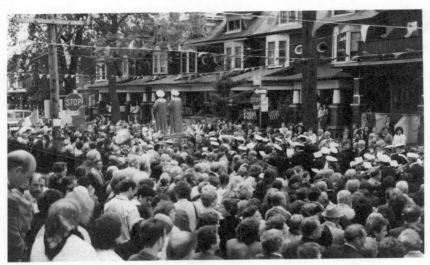

FIGURE 2.7 Crowd at the Toronto feast, 1992.

or relatives. The procession can take up to two hours; it moves slowly but without stopping, in a giant circle, south on Grace, west for a block on Dundas, north up to College, turning east for several blocks before heading back south and then west to the church. Police stop traffic on the major arteries. The route falls in the shadow of the Toronto Hospital (formerly Toronto Western Hospital)—a temple to modern science—where I had spent two years during my student days and residency and my first husband had been chief medical resident (Figure 2.8). In the evening light, the Toronto saints can be admired with the hospital and the CN Tower over their shoulders.

I asked Father Paonessa about the relationship of the statues to the celebration. Perhaps he sensed some suspicion over the commandment against worshipping images; however, he welcomed the question and explained that the statues were necessary, not as idols, but as the proper set for a splendid opera. They were part of Italian tradition. They had been the gift of a family in the parish. Father Ralph denied his own influence and credited the festival's existence to the keen and intense devotion of the donor family and its successful continuity to the tremendous social functions it fills. Having had small contact with his exuberant charm, I found this modest statement difficult to believe. But then he offered a surprising observation that hard feelings arose as people in Utica, New York, complained about the loss of Toronto pilgrims who used to attend a feast there and seemed to have "stolen" the idea.[72] He urged me to talk to the donor family, assuring me that they would be willing.

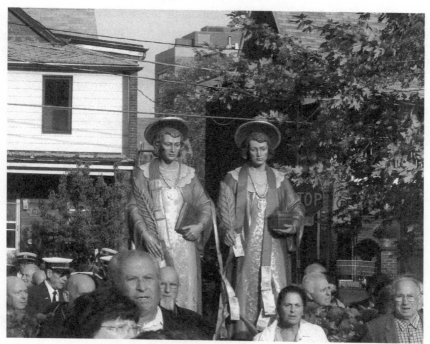

FIGURE 2.8 Procession with Toronto Hospital in distance, 2010. Photo by Jessica Duffin Wolfe.

Driven though I was to find out about the arrival of the saints, I was conscious that my quest intruded into a private, spiritual space. Unable to bring myself to call, I wrote a letter of explanation, but received no reply. I sent another announcing that I would soon telephone to request a meeting when I was next in Toronto. On the appointed day, I mustered up my courage and called. Mercifully, the person who replied seemed not to be surprised. In rough Italian and English with two unknown but friendly people, a time was fixed for the following day. My obsession with Cosmas and Damian was causing me to do things I would normally strive to avoid. I took Anita with me. Friendship and location were good support, but it was her courage and professional skills that I needed most.

On a cold February afternoon, we found the modest house on Dundas Street, not far from Saint Francis Church. Before knocking, we stamped snow from our boots and placed them neatly on the mat in the enclosed porch. A strong, square-ish man in his sixties opened the door; he did not look pleased to see us. I tried to explain about the phone call the previous day. He shook his head, either uncomprehending or unwilling to comprehend. We tried

gesturing with our hands and saying "santi medici." His wife appeared behind
him, looking no more welcoming. Wanting the painful moment to end, I
offered to go away. That suggestion brought immediate acquiescence, but I
could tell Anita was displeased with my capitulation. We stooped to put
on our boots. The stern man went away, but the woman stood in the open
doorway, watching.

As soon as our boots were done up and we were set to go, she said quietly,
"Wann'a caf'?"

"No. No thanks. It's okay," I said, heading for the steps.

"Yes!" said Anita, grabbing my arm and looking cross. "We want a caf'!"
"Are you crazy?" the psychiatrist hissed at me. "She wants to talk to us!" Off
came our boots again.

We went to the kitchen; the husband did not reappear, but adult daughter
Mary, who spoke perfect English, came downstairs to help communicate. She
seemed to have been expecting us, but explained that her parents were upset
because she was getting a divorce.

Ersilia Jannetta (Mrs. Di Gregorio) came to Canada in 1953 from Campobasso province of south central Italy.[73] She retired after forty years of working
as a babysitter. Aptly, it seems, her parents were a midwife and a former monk.
The monk had been summoned from his monastery to the village of his birth
to tend his dying mother. He needed help with her intimate care, and the
midwife was engaged. When the monk's mother died, he did not return to
the monastery but married the midwife instead. The couple had twelve children. Ersilia went with her large family to many religious events, including
the Cosmas and Damian festival in Isernia. They were, however, devoted to
all the saints. When Ersilia came to Canada she missed the santi medici most
of all and vowed to bring them to Toronto.

After many years, Ersilia and her husband had gathered the funds to purchase the statues and air-transport them from Rome. The family participates
in the procession every year; they also help in the decoration of the church.
On some feast days, Ersilia and her daughter stand at the top of the church
steps while the statues return, as if to greet them.

Ersilia showed me the tangible evidence of the first Toronto miracle: a
carefully wrapped cane and written testimonial of a woman healed of a
knee ailment and spared surgical amputation. In leaving her cane with
Ersilia, the woman said, "The saints help me, I help the saints." Ersilia said
that modern medicine, doctors, and hospitals were good, but they did
not provide hope; the saints brought hope to everyone when the medicine ran out.

Ersilia had been to Utica, New York, she told me, but she did not enjoy the long bus ride and did not understand why the santi medici could not come to Canada too.

More Theories: Mythology, Psychology, Sociology, and Twins

Now I knew the proximate cause of the feast day celebration in Toronto—a motivated family and an immigrant tradition. I began to wonder if some parts of Italy had venerated the medical saints more than others. Still clinging to the idea that they might be related to Castor and Pollux, I thought that perhaps those places venerating the saints could somehow be connected to the ancient cult of the Dioscuri or to the even older Indo-European twins.

The majority of Italians in Toronto had migrated from southern Italy—a place often referred to as Magna Graecia because it had been settled by Greeks long before the rise of the Roman empire. Perhaps the Greeks had been more enthusiastic about the Dioscuri, or maybe their version had been less militaristic and more medical than the Roman. Little in the literature supported either hypothesis. However, Pierre Julien had shown clearly that the most elaborate feast day celebrations to Cosmas and Damian were concentrated in southern Italy and Sicily.[74] Eighty percent or more of Italians who live in Toronto originated in southern Italy or Sicily.[75]

In any case, the conversation with Ersilia suggested that the saints were filling important functions in the present. I needed some theoretical help from mythology, sociology, anthropology, and perhaps even psychology.[76] It seemed most obvious to start with the twin angle.

For specialists in mythology, twins reflect natural dualities—good and bad, life and death, sickness and health. They seemed to be everywhere. Either they were handed down from one culture to another in that genealogy of traditions described earlier, or twin deities were discovered repeatedly but independently as a collective understanding of experience, called "universal Dioscurism." A wider phenomenon than the inherited, genealogical variety, universal Dioscurism implies that twin gods may be repeatedly found and venerated for psychological reasons in cultures that have nothing to do with each other.[77] Cosmas and Damian would therefore be simply one more manifestation of a globally distributed human proclivity.

The idea of multiple discoveries implied that the divine twins filled a distinct role, a perceived function that was somehow timeless. Could it be that all peoples eventually develop an actual *need* for divine twins—and how could that work?

A psychoanalytic theory holds that myths function to preserve social and psychological stability. The powerful, natural events of birth, life, illness, and death threaten moral, social, and psychological order. Twins represent fertility, an excess of vitality, and, in a sense, rebirth. They may also signify the triumph of life-giving order over the chaos of death. They are super-vital; when they heal, the life-sustaining properties are all the stronger.[78] Like some anthropomorphized Yin and Yang, mythic twins may rehearse natural dualities in human existence: sickness and health; life and death, or in medical existence: diagnosis and nondiagnosis; therapeutic success and failure.

While the psychological theory addressed the *causes* of the twin deities, a sociological view addresses the actual *functions* that such divinities could fill in a social context. Without necessarily believing in the divinity of the gods, sociologists have long recognized religion as a powerful force for social cohesion, order, advice, and comfort. Emile Durkheim made early contributions to the field by emphasizing that religion entailed community. It can bind people to their culture, sway political and health behaviors, and sustain migrants far from home.[79] On this view, then, Cosmas and Damian could console and unite as reminders of national traditions within an uprooted community—Father Ralph implied as much. They might also be operating as divine healers, filling some kind of role in health provision for people who value their medical attributes.

The existence of twin deities who cannot be linked to Indo-European origins supports the psychological and sociological views against a genealogical theory. For example, the Egyptians venerated Isis and Osiris, one living, one dead, brother and sister gods of medicine, healing, death, and afterlife. African tribes were said to have a pair of twin gods whose rivalry might be said to reflect inner conflicts.[80] Amerindian and Japanese mythologies also recognize powerful sibling dyads.[81] Some cultures mistrusted double births, but that anxiety also fed into their mystical roles.

My First Paper on the Saints, 1992

The thread I was pulling on simply got longer and longer, and more tangled. Unable to leave the topic alone and having spent so much time reading and thinking about it, I decided to propose a paper for the annual meeting of the Canadian Society for the History of Medicine in June 1992. This small but friendly group of historians, doctors, librarians, nurses, and students gathers once a year to discuss our current research. I was hoping for advice and direction. It felt fraudulent to be calling this curiosity "research," but doing so legitimized obsession. To my amazement the proposal was accepted.

I prepared a twenty-minute talk to outline the questions, and to situate the observations in light of the four theoretical explanations, all of which seemed to make some sense with respect to the Toronto celebration: a simple diffusion model, the genealogical theory, the psychoanalytic model, and the sociological model of religious function.

The diffusion theory enjoyed the most actual evidence as an explanation for the coming of Cosmas and Damian from Italy to Toronto. The French have an expression for moving house: *"transférer ses pénates."* Literally, it means "to move one's household gods." Diffusion encapsulates that idea perfectly. Ersilia herself referred to the celebration in Isernia as a place where she had honored the saints that she later transported from Italy. The Canadian form of the celebration presumably related to those back home.

I argued that several aspects of the doctor saints supported the wider genealogical theory. First, pagan temples often became churches; churches to the doctor saints were sometimes built in the defunct healing temples, or Asklepeia.[82] Second, some of Cosmas and Damian's cures suggested the ancient rite of incubation, as if the providers may have changed but the treatments did not. Third, the practice of leaving votive objects was adopted by the Christians from pagan traditions by at least the fourth century AD and continues today at all Christian shrines.[83] Fourth, the saintly attributes and functions of Cosmas and Damian can indeed be linked to the Dioscuri, if only because of the proximity of their respective temples in the Roman Forum, both close to the Juturna fountain of miraculous cures.[84]

Without choosing one view over another, I brought in other possible explanations, including the psychological theory for possible "causes" of deities as twins and the sociological model about function, peculiar not only on this cult, but to religious healing in general. The saints could be active healers in the communities that venerated them. I liked the paper but was afraid of what colleagues might say.

The meeting was held at the University of Prince Edward Island in Charlottetown. The gathering was small—perhaps forty people. The society is so diverse that hostile questions are a rarity. To my horror, two famous historians slipped into the back row just as I began to speak. But the talk went well and comments were pointed but polite. Perhaps, someone suggested, this Toronto feast was simply identical to all other Italian immigrant celebrations. Could I demonstrate anything peculiar to Cosmas and Damian? It was all well and good to emphasize the donor family's relationship to Italy, but what was the role of Utica, New York, and were those American celebrants of Italian origin too? How could I prove which of the theories was most relevant to the project? Can this work really be called history? And what did it contribute to my practice as a physician? The last question came from one of the famous historians. I had no answer.

Later in the traditional beer tent, I spoke with the two brainy classicists of the group who had been silent during the meeting, Paul Potter and Gilles Maloney. I worried that they scorned my bumbling onto their ancient turf with the genealogical theory and my total lack of Greek. Perhaps the project struck them as sophomoric and derivative. But they seemed indifferent to my incursion, as if any right-minded scholar must always touch base with the ancients, however poorly, before clearing her throat. They agreed that the best part had been the Toronto feast: "Now *that's* interesting!"

At the hotel out on the beach, sociologist Joe Lella was curious and encouraging. He seemed not in the least troubled by my lack of credentials in cultural anthropology; he gave me references to sociological studies of Italians in New York City.

It was a benediction to continue. This obsessive curiosity had officially become "research." I went to the Toronto feast in 1992, spoke to another priest, and shot several rolls of film.

The Utica Celebration

Obviously, something had been happening in upstate New York that was directly related to the founding of the Toronto feast, and, as the Charlottetown audience pointed out, I had ignored it. Perhaps Toronto owed far more to Utica than it did to Italy—and maybe the feast in Utica was not Italian at all.

Deacon William (Bill) Dischiavo of Saint Anthony of Padua parish in Utica readily supplied the history on the telephone and in print.[85] Established by Italian immigrants in 1912, a year after the founding of their church, the Utica feast was modeled on the same celebration in their home town of Alberobello, in the southern Italian region of Puglia. Bill's grandmother, Signora Dischiavo (née Gerardi), was born in Foggia, and came to the United States in 1904 with her parents, three sisters, and one brother. The family worked in the cotton mills. No special attention was given to the medical saints in

Foggia, but Signora Dischiavo was deeply devoted to them and to the patron of the parish from her late teens until her death at age ninety in 1983. Bill remembers her intense prayers during a particularly wet celebration in the 1950s when he was seven or eight years old. It had rained all night and the ground was sodden; his grandmother knelt in the mud praying fervently for his older brother who was severely afflicted with polio. The boy lived with only minor sequelae.

Since its inception, the Utica feast has taken the form of one or more masses and two or more processions. From the late 1940s, additional services were held outdoors to accommodate the large crowds. Three masses comprise the full event: one for the sick on Friday, another on Saturday evening followed by the candlelit procession through the neighborhood streets, and a third on Sunday morning, also followed by a midday procession. The Sunday event is festive and more secular. Each year two adolescent boys take part, dressed in costumes as the saints (Figure 2.9). Representatives of several fraternities also participate, traveling from places up to eight hours away, including Toronto. Images of the saints abound, on banners at private homes and as statues in or near the church.

Several sets of statues of the medical saints can be found in Utica. When the originals were destroyed by fire in 1947, a collection was taken to bring new statues from Rome. But the immigrants from Alberobello

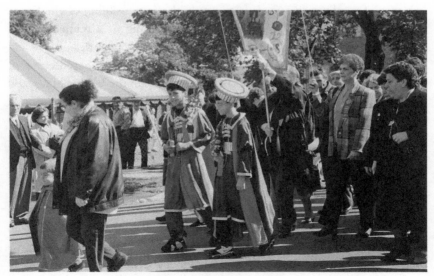

FIGURE 2.9 Boys dressed as the saints, Utica, NY, 1996.

were disappointed with the new statues of saints that seemed "too young" and "beardless." This set remains in a chapel inside the church to the right of the altar. Another collection was taken for a new pair of statues ordered specifically to resemble the ones in their Italian hometown. Larger than life, these two wooden effigies feature red and green robes and prominent, dark beards; they are the ones used in the processions. Unlike those in Toronto, which share a podium, these statues are separate. During the feast days, they wear cloth capes—Cosmas in red, Damian in green. In inclement weather, they don clear, plastic raincoats, with the help of Deacon Dischiavo. All the statues—inside and outside—are festooned with ribbons of money.

To accommodate the large crowds, the parish rents costly tents each year. A permanent outdoor altar was first erected in 1950 with its own statues, but it was reconstructed in 1984, and the statues of the original altar were buried in the new foundation. At that time, yet another set of bearded statues in pure white Carrera marble was commissioned from Rome. On the back of the outdoor altar is the double-winged caduceus, originally of the pagan god Mercury (not Aesculapius), used as a symbol by the American Medical Association—a wonderful juxtaposition of religious and professional symbolism, complete with cultural slippage.

More statues of the medical saints can be found in a chapel on Utica's Kossuth Avenue. Apparently, a conflict had arisen in the 1940s among the organizers of the Utica celebration. The chapel, begun in the 1950s, was the response of a splinter group. It is currently the responsibility of the Saints Cosmo and Damiano Congregation, Inc. According to a mimeographed flyer, it is "a simple holy place made elaborate by the memories of love and devotion and the five and ten cent contributions of a very special group of local Barese, pilgrims, and believers from all corners of the United States and Canada." The site was revived in the 1970s and a panoramic wall painting of Alberobello was completed in 1985. Pilgrims now go to both the church and the chapel as components of the complete tour. Few of those involved in the original rift are still living; consequently, the reasons for the rift are forgotten and surveillance in the chapel is lax: one year all the monetary donations left there were stolen.[86]

Deacon Dischiavo claims that Utica has the largest feast for the medical saints in North America. In the 1960s, attendance lagged and "only fourteen or fifteen busloads" of pilgrims would attend. During the early 1990s, however, ten to twelve thousand pilgrims attended, arriving in seventy or eighty busses.

For the celebration in September 1994, hotels as far as forty-five minutes away were fully booked by early July. The city benefits from the influx of visitors, but it does not contribute to the costs, which must be covered by collections at the church and donations at the feast day. When asked to account for the recent resurgence in popularity of the Utica celebration, Deacon Dischiavo immediately identified the leadership of the immigrants who courageously built a life in a new land, without forgetting the traditions of home. He believes that people are motivated by disillusionment with modern ways to "go back to their roots" and return to spirituality, a trend that had been noticed in the media at that time.[87] Like Father Paonessa, Father Dischiavo described the social and economic functions served by the celebration and influx of visitors: traditional foods, decoration of homes, sale of religious objects, music and dancing, and the chance to greet old friends. He is unhappy about, but resigned to the presence of, street vendors of T-shirts, aprons, and cloth bags who set up as close to the church as possible, turning a tidy profit without contributing to expenses.

I asked if there had been miracles. Deacon Dischiavo replied that his brother's healing from polio may have been owing to the intercession of the saints through the prayers of his grandmother; however, he admitted that he has not asked his brother's own opinion. Other cures are inferred from the discarded casts and crutches left behind or offerings of gold, now worth an amount so considerable that they must be kept in the church safe. Two Utica physicians participate enthusiastically in the procession. But Dischiavo cautioned that the healings are as much spiritual as physical.

When asked why Torontonians still come to Utica, Dischiavo explained that approximately thirty years ago, in an effort to promote the Utica celebration, he placed an advertisement in a Toronto newspaper. That year, a single bus left Toronto to join the other twenty to thirty buses traveling to Utica from elsewhere. The next year, Torontonians filled three buses; the following year, fifteen. The Toronto priest, Father Paonessa confirmed these figures saying that demand in Toronto in the late 1980s would have filled forty or fifty busses—two thousand people. After a few years of making the tiring journey, people in Toronto thought it might be easier to celebrate at home. Overworked and not lacking for pilgrims, Deacon Dischiavo did not display the "hard feelings" that had been described in Toronto. As for why many Torontonians would continue to make the trip to Utica when they could now celebrate at home, he replied, "People want the sacrifice of pilgrimage." "The journey," he added, "is part of the prayer."

The Second Paper on Cosmas and Damian

A pattern was emerging: immigrants transport their saints for "use" in their new homes as spiritual and physical support.

Having heard the talk in Charlottetown, my friend, Gina Feldberg, extended an invitation to York University's Health and Society seminars in March 1993. This was a fabulous opportunity because her unit included not only social historians like herself, but also sociologists and anthropologists. I was hoping for suggestions about those theories that had seemed so promising in terms of explanation, but too amorphous in terms of research. Perhaps these scholars knew how to direct work toward answering the new questions that the theories had sparked. Franca Iacovetta attended the small gathering. Her new book, *Such Hardworking People*, on the Italians in Toronto, had been a touchstone for situating the feast-day celebration.[88]

The small group sat around a large table in a windowless room while I presented the ideas that I had been playing with to explain the feast day. Yes, diffusion, and now possibly rivalry with or imitation of Utica, were the most obvious explanations for why the feast was celebrated in Toronto. But I could not lose sight of the origins in a more remote past, nor did I want to relinquish the idea of the medical saints filling functions in the present.

The York scholars were friendly, polite, and encouraging. But they seemed noncommittal about the theories—preferring none, and not reacting badly to any. At the end, Franca stated the obvious.

"You have to ask them."

"What do you mean? Ask the pilgrims at the celebrations?"

"Yes," she said. "It's all well and good to hypothesize on grand theories about the roles that those saints may be filling in their lives. But the only way to find out what the saints are doing there is to ask them."

She was right. This "research" was morphing in scary directions. No longer could it be called history. Technically speaking, it was sociology—and I had no credentials.

In September 1994, I attended the Utica feast, taking my Jewish husband and two children along. Ten-year-old Jessica especially liked the candlelight procession. At seventeen, Joshua was embarrassed but patient, and he didn't complain about the cannoli. We watched the activities, the masses, and the partying with good food and dancing. Busy though he was, Deacon Dischiavo welcomed us and introduced several people who had been marking the feast all their lives.

Franca's advice haunted me. Could I ever walk up to complete strangers at a religious event and demand to know what they were doing there? And if I did muster that kind of courage, would the answers be meaningful?

The most sobering discovery of that weekend was Bill Dischiavo's casual remark about another, smaller feast taking place at Church of the Most Precious Blood in Manhattan. How many such celebrations did these saints enjoy? And if Franca's surveying was to be done, must it include them all? I had to go looking for Cosmas and Damian wherever they could be found; and I had to start talking to pilgrims systematically. Although I was not intending to focus exclusively on the celebrations, the best way to find devotees was at the feasts.

Having officially become "research," this project was perverse: it could be advanced on only one day of the year.

THE DOCTOR SAINTS came to Toronto in 1987. Essential factors in their appearance were a devout donor who had emigrated from Italy, a rival, older celebration in another city, and a perception that modern medicine was failing. But colleagues and the scholarly literature reminded me that the advent of the santi medici to Toronto might be just a tiny manifestation of larger patterns that apply to the movement of religious custom in any time and place. Those theories about patterns seemed plausible, but were they all relevant? To discover what Cosmas and Damian were doing in Toronto, I had to ask the people whom they served.

3

Talking to Pilgrims in the New World

*I do believe I begin to grasp the nature of miracles! For
would it be a miracle, if there was any reason for it?
Miracles have nothing to do with reason. Miracles contra-
dict reason, overturn reason, make game of reason, they
strike clean across mere human deserts, and deliver and
save where they will. If they made sense, they would not be
miracles.*

—BROTHER CADFAEL, *Ellis Peters, A Morbid Taste for Bones, 1977, ch. 11*

The Third Paper

Every year, an academic receives dozens of announcements for conferences
that have nothing to do with her own research. We pass them along to colleagues and students who might be interested, or toss them in the recycle box.
Once in a while, they speak to us personally. Shortly after the visit to York
University and with the suggestions of Gina Feldberg and Franca Iacovetta
still ringing in my ears, the arrival of one such flyer caught my eye. It came
from the Institute for Cultural History in Amsterdam announcing a conference on "Healing, Magic, and Belief in Europe, 15th to 20th Centuries. New
Perspectives."

Granted I was working on North America, not Europe, but I knew enough
to connect the feasts to Italy and France; more importantly, I needed help.
"New Perspectives" sounded just right. So I sent off a proposal, not caring
much whether it would be approved or not, although acceptance would permit an application for financial support for the trip. If it were to be rejected, I
might attend the conference anyway, simply to meet the medical historians
who make this type of research their stock in trade. The proposal was accepted, and the pseudo-project was slowly gathering more dignity than it
seemed to deserve.

More surprises were in store. The conference papers were to be precircu-
lated. Divided into large panels, we would each have just ten minutes to
"speak to" our work before a general discussion around a theme. Ideally, all the
delegates would read the submissions in advance of the meeting. Consequently, a huge binder of papers arrived just as I was leaving. I spent the long
flight to Amsterdam reading through these essays and feeling more and more
like an outsider. The organizers had lured an international array of scholars
interested in unorthodox healing practices, especially witchcraft, magic, and
folk healing. Despite the title and time frame in the original call for papers,
few of the contributions addressed orthodox religion or regular medicine;
nor did they feature anything more recent than the eighteenth century. It
promised to be a gathering of a club to which I did not belong. And it meant
I needed to learn more about magic.

But the conference was friendly and the organizers had planned well.
They chose Woudshoten, a woodland retreat at Zeist, near Utrecht south of
Amsterdam—"the second largest forest in the Netherlands," people kept
telling us with big grins. To a Canadian, the several-acre preserve seemed
more like a medium-sized city park. But the misty autumn light made for
exquisite morning walks, and socializing was easy, if not enforced, because
there was nowhere else to go. Outings were arranged by bus over the flat, ca-
nalled landscape to Boerhaave Museum for the history of science in Leiden
and to the sixteenth-century Witches' Weigh House in Oudewater with its
"scale" for "diagnosing" and judging witches. Most women so tested were
found innocent. Indeed, some delegates, with their goth-like dress, hair, jew-
elry, and makeup might have failed the witch test.

My paper was called "Saints Cosmas and Damian of Toronto: Origin and
Meaning of the Medical Cult of Divine Twins." No one attacked it. Mostly it
was ignored. Several people took me at my word when I said that I wanted suggestions for future directions. The intrepid organizer, Marijke Gijswijt-Hofstra,
dismissed my fear that the work did not belong, and she endorsed Franca's notion of interviews. Stylish and funny, the English specialist in folklore, Gillian
Bennett, was surrounded by admirers during the breaks and meals. Specializing
in ghost stories, she showed how legends can be powerful sources for cultural
history. Her paper had been on the meaning of the "breast serpent," a recurring
tale related to health. Just such a miraculous cure had appeared in the tales of
Cosmas and Damian. Gillian's research suggested that not only the twinliness
of the saints, but also their deeds, could belong to ancient oral traditions. Her
work seemed enviously delightful—so far removed from medicine and history
in that her sources didn't even pretend to be true. Wietse de Boer cheerfully

offered comments and Ineke van Wetering provided references to anthropological work on twin deities in Africa. They also pointed out literature of the "how
to" variety to help with the interviews that I had yet to conduct. Several scholars
whom I met at Zeist are still my friends—Hilary Marland, Frank Huisman, and
Enrique Perdiguero. We all look back fondly on what we call the "witch conference in the woods." It was magic.

Indeed, magic was the biggest surprise. These scholars were confident in
their understanding of what it was—belief in supernatural powers that could
be manipulated by humans within various traditions. But my miracles were
the result of divine intervention, which is also supernatural, following a
human appeal. It was not clear to me—and it still isn't—how exactly magical
healing differed from religious or medical healing.

I spent a long time trying to decipher the philosophical and theological
definitions of "miracle" and "magic"; "religion" and "medicine." The literature
was confusing. Newer definitions of "miracle" are said to dispense with the
supernatural and the criterion of defying natural law to emphasize instead
divine healing and the unanticipated; some definitions appeal to logic and
semiology.[1] Since Vatican II and, perhaps, in acceptance of this new, "natural-
istic" view of miracle, it seems that the church has tried to distance itself from
popular miracles and healing in particular.[2] Yet others express concern about
this trend away from the miraculous, because we need to make space for "signs
of the presence of God."[3] Elsewhere, church officials have stressed the extent
to which miracles used for the rite of canonization are scientifically scruti-
nized and endorsed.[4] Those cases would imply that the word "miracle" can be
used only after official investigations permit it.

In my search to understand the differences in meaning, I found that several
great scholars have attempted to distinguish between the workings of medicine, magic, and miracle, and they remind us that the meaning of miracles
kept changing.[5] Magic was supposed to be condemned by Christians. But as
medical historian Owsei Temkin observed, "principle was one thing and practice another"; from the earliest times, "it was not always easy to draw the line
between legitimate and magical remedies."[6] For sociologist Émile Durkheim,
religion involved community, unlike magic, which was a provider-client
dyad.[7] But now I doubt that anyone has made these distinctions successfully
with respect to other people, let alone other cultures—because no one wishes
to claim magic for themselves. The fuzzy boundaries between these categories
are falsely sharpened by doctors, priests, philosophers, and, indeed, by historians of medicine, who tend to focus on one or another category, as if it were
distinct from the others.[8] To a believer of one faith, other religious practices

are magical. To a confident physician, all other forms of practice, including religion, alternative, and past medicines, are magical.

For medical historians, magic was once portrayed as the first step along continuum through religion to science—a trend reified by an older generation who saw the magic of "primitive" medicine steadily swept away by the march of science. Recent scholarship has tried to avoid this positivistic, self-congratulatory perspective through the conceptual vehicles of social function and placebo effect.[9] Some, especially nurses, go so far as to acknowledge, if not recommend, the value of some rituals in current practice.[10] But no medically trained healers in our time choose to call themselves "magicians." Nor is it a word that the religious would apply to their priests. Even the self-identified, professional magicians of today are known to all not as healers or wizards, but as kindly deceivers of children.

Magic is a word readily applied to the "story" told by someone else, from another culture, place, or time—Merlin and Harry Potter.[11] Since no patients, no pilgrims, and no practitioners in our time would choose to apply the word to themselves, I concluded that "magic" should not be equated with "miracle" as it is understood by religious people.

Now it was time to design those surveys in preparation for the feast days in 1995.

The Surveys

Sociological methods long turned on the value of numbers as quantitative evidence, but in the postmodern era, attempts were made to uncover qualitative information too.[12] Obviously both were relevant to my questions. I examined a variety of other surveys of popular religion for inspiration.[13] Years later, a reader of the manuscript for this book would complain that I had rejected in-depth interviews with devotees, and opted instead for a somewhat quantitative approach; she or he qualified his observation with the words, "easy to say in hindsight." Whether or not it was a conscious decision, I chose a method that could allow brief but meaningful encounters, hoping that it would not be too intrusive and that the random selection of people would be representative of the whole. Rather than wishing to probe the inner workings of individual faith, I was more interested in the social and medical role (if any) of the medical saints in our time.

All advice emphasized that the fewer the questions asked, the better. I designed a simple, one-page questionnaire with a paragraph on the back to explain who I was and what I was doing. The questions needed to explore the theories—Where had the saints come from? What attributes were most important—their twinliness? Their medicine? Were they actually working for the people who came to celebrate them? If so, how? I also needed to know something about the people themselves, such as age, origins, and home.

One concern did influence the design of the questionnaire. I worried that this project would simply morph into a sociological study of Italian immigrant culture—something that had already been done several times by sociologists and anthropologists far better equipped for the task.[14] I was interested mostly in Cosmas and Damian, but I had to admit that their celebrations were not unique and could typify all Italian festivals; moreover, exactly the same answers about their function could come from devotees of other saints too. But pragmatics reigned. If I wanted to know what people were thinking about the medical saints and the reasons for their devotion all year long, the only way to locate those involved was to target the pilgrims at the feast-day rites; however, I had to remember that those distracting, festive trappings were not my main focus. Furthermore, all saints are invoked for healing at one time or another. Consequently, on some level, all saints are medical. Until shown otherwise by someone else, Cosmas and Damian could possibly represent them all.

Just before the Holland conference, I had been joined by a new colleague in medical history: Terrie Romano. Born in Canada of parents from Italy, Terrie had Mediterranean verve and a keen sense of the outrageous. With her dissertation on a British physiologist, she was an expert on nineteenth-century medical science; but her latest research addressed how botanists described carnivorous plants as if they were voracious, predatory women. Terrie liked my saints project. With her grandmother's help, she translated the questionnaire into Italian. Her grandmother too found the project interesting and sent a message that I should not be afraid of asking people about their devotions. This kindness helped.

Any research with "human subjects" requires ethics approval, and I had to submit the questionnaire to my medical-school colleagues for consideration and endorsement. Just as the quest had become "research," this modest questionnaire was now called a "survey instrument." Consent was implied by a willingness to complete the form or reply to its questions in person. With no plans to test medicines or use needles, approval came quickly.

During my 1995 sabbatical, I went back to France in order to finish researching and revising my dissertation for what would become a book on the stethoscope. But I could not go away for long because my husband was working and the children were in school. No excuse remained for getting on with those interviews. To engage with the maximum number of pilgrims, it was necessary to

The Survey Instrument

1. How many times have you come to the celebration for SS Cosmas and Damian at the Church of XXX? (circle the best answer)

   1   2–5   6–10   11–15   16–20   21–25   more_____

2. Why do you come? (circle as many as you like, and feel free to add more)

   tradition in family

   special fondness for SS Cosmas and Damian

   friends

   go to all the celebrations in this parish

   other_____

3. Is it special or important for you that SS Cosmas and Damian are twins?

   yes   not really   don't know/never thought about it

4. Is it special or important for you that SS Cosmas and Damian are doctors?

   yes   not really   don't know/never thought about it

5. Are you aware of any miracles by the intercession of SS Cosmas and Damian?

   yes (if you don't mind, please describe briefly below or on back)   no

6. Are you aware of any other SS Cosmas and Damian celebrations in the USA, Canada, or Italy? If yes, where_____

7. How old are you?

   less than 20 yrs   20–39 yrs   40–59 yrs   60–79 yrs   80 or more

8. Are you

   female   male?

9. Where are your own roots or those of your parents?

   If Italy, what town_____   other_____

10. From how far away have you come for the celebration?

   same city   nearby   other (place/ km or miles)_____

11. Would you be willing to talk to a student about SS Cosmas and Damian?

   yes (please name address & phone on back, or on separate page)

   no (that's quite OK)

travel to as many of the feast-day celebrations as possible. The crunch came from the difficulty of trying to be in two or more places at once. Mercifully, parishes might pick different days either side of September 27th to mark the feast.

I began with the crowds in Toronto (Figure 3.1). To avoid actually having to talk to people, I entertained the idea of leaving the forms lying around with

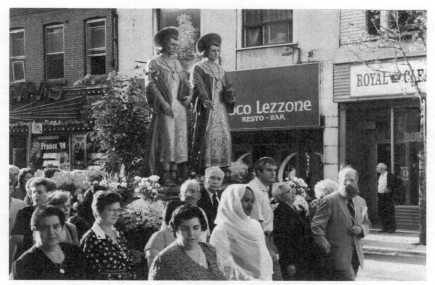

FIGURE 3.1 Toronto procession on College Street, 1998. Photo by Ian Billingsley.

a few small pencils. A drop box could collect the completed forms. With the permission of the Toronto priest, I scattered the sheets of paper over the pews of Saint Francis of Assisi church well before the congregation began to assemble for its feast-day mass. Slowly, the congregation began to fill the church. They were mostly working-class citizens with tanned faces and rough hands, decked out in their Sunday best. It quickly became obvious that they were ignoring my survey instruments—sitting on them, crumpling them, sliding them out of the way with barely a glance. The clever plan was failing. Appalled, I realized that I must talk to these strangers or wait yet another year. When the mass was over and the procession about to begin, I tried approaching a few people milling about in the crowd.

"Excuse me. May I ask you a few questions?" Most stopped, were friendly, and tried to understand. It was easiest to make contact in person and show them the questions in writing. I could record their responses. The majority preferred Terrie's Italian version. One woman grew angry; offended by my intrusion on her spiritual endeavor, she shoved me aside. A slim, elderly lady smiled as she watched that small drama. With her coiffed blond hair, gold brocade coat, and matching pumps and purse, she seemed withdrawn and wealthier than the others. She lurked in the background, but did not volunteer to take the survey. Later, as the procession set off and the crowd thinned, she stepped forward, I hoped, to answer the questions. But instead she said,

"I know what you are. *Una giornalista*!" Franca may have been right that it was important to talk to the pilgrims, but I hated doing it.

I drove the four hours to Utica alone this time. The Howard Johnson hotel where we had stayed the year before had lost my reservation and was full, but the staff helped locate a room in a modest motel not too far away. I would camp there for two nights, observe the whole event, and try to talk to as many people as possible. Bill Dischiavo was very busy but seemed pleased that I'd returned; he had given permission for the questions in advance. Once again an enormous crowd had gathered. Over two whole days, the people spent a lot of time simply enjoying food, music, and dancing while waiting for the masses and procession (Figure 3.2). The church ran a cafeteria in the basement and various concessions were selling food in the church yard. The influx brought with it a little burst of prosperity: the local bakers claimed that it was their best week of the year.

The interviews were easier in Utica than they had been in Toronto; most could handle English even if they did not prefer it. But the comfort wasn't only owing to language—the atmosphere was more relaxed; lingering and making new friends seemed de rigueur. Chatting with a group at the dining tables would attract notice from others, who would wave me over to talk to them too. Some seemed eager to comply and reminisce; others introduced friends with spectacular stories.

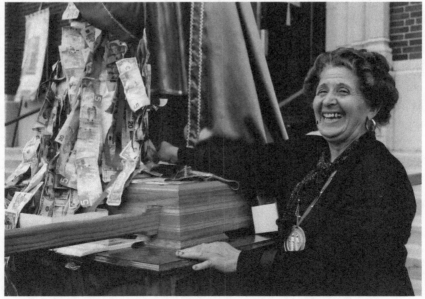

FIGURE 3.2 Catherine Putruele pinning Canadian money to statues, Utica, NY, 2003.

The clarinetist in the local band—a man of at least sixty years—had been saved from diphtheria at the age of four, after his parents appealed to Saints Cosmas and Damian. Several told tales of family members who had been ill and had recovered after seeing visions of the saints. Four young women who were not of Italian origin were attending for the first time; one of them suffered from a chronic illness and they seemed embarrassed to admit that they were "checking it out" from a medical angle. A radiant young widow in black chided me about the miracle question—saying that her miracle was the gift of life and her children. She was from Toronto. "Why come all the way to Utica when you can celebrate at home?" I asked her. She smiled, responding, "This celebration is older and more authentic. It's more original and so it's better."

I left Utica with many completed questionnaires.

Cosmas and Damian of Québec

Any hope of tracking down all the sites that now venerated the medical saints was beginning to fade. On the one hand, it seemed that a numberless series of small centers each hosted subtle variations upon the theme; I could not visit them all. A proper appreciation of each event meant an in-person visit, and, given the calendar, only one or two could be accomplished each year. On the other hand, it seemed that these celebrations were decidedly Italian, having more to do with nostalgia for homeland and family tradition than with medicine and its history.

Sites of pilgrimage and thaumaturgic healing are numerous in Canada, especially in Québec, but the literature on the subject did not mention the medical saints.[15] Nevertheless, scholarship on the nature of the sites of devotion and the miracles attributed to the saints shows a preponderance of physical healings.[16] In the fall of 1995, I looked at the index of a map of Québec. At least two towns were named Saint-Côme, and another two Saint-Damien, all four situated off the beaten track on either side of the Saint Lawrence River, each with a population of around 2,000. The two north of the great river were located relatively close to each other, just south of the beautiful park of Mont Tremblant. Between them lay the village of Ste. Émélie-de-l'Énergie, whose intriguing name is unexplained but may commemorate the verve of a settler's wife or the courage of hardy pioneers. Finding scant information about these villages in any library, I decided to drive there, hoping to find answers to my questions about their names.

It was October 1995 and a Québec referendum on separation was brewing. As I drove north out of Montreal, signs favoring "Oui!" in favor of separation

greatly outnumbered those for "Non!" How would I be received? I booked
into the only motel in town. Saint-Côme Lanaudière was geared toward receiving visitors for winter sports, but things were very quiet in October. The
church was a vast, white, wooden structure; its doors were locked. At the *mai-
rie*, the reception was friendly. No priest lived in town, but everyone urged me
to visit the village historian, Mademoiselle Eulalie Riopel, whose quaint gray
house with a scooped Québec roof nestled on the edge of town by the river.

Petite, articulate Eulalie had grown up in the village and collected anec-
dotes of its history in immaculate folders. Now in her seventies, she had an
encyclopedic memory and her classification system allowed her to find whatever she was looking for.

I learned from Eulalie that settlers came to Saint-Côme around 1862, with
the first priest arriving in 1867. She assured me that Monseigneur Ignace
Bourget, the famous archbishop of Montreal, had designated the patron saint
of this town and that of its sister, Saint-Damien, because they were so far from
physicians and hospitals. Therefore, the fledgling towns needed the added
medical support of doctor-saints. The Saint-Côme church opened in 1886.
Eulalie remembered that once beautiful murals of the lives of the saints decorated its walls, but they had been painted over many years ago in an "improvement scheme" of which she did not approve. She doubted that anyone had
kept photos of the murals; no particular events were held on the feast day, and
she thought few people nowadays realized that Côme was the twin of Damien,
or that he was a doctor.

Saint-Damien-de-Brandon was more agricultural and lay on a low hillside
overlooking a shallow valley. A good, local history belonged to the McGill
University library and I corresponded with its author, Thérèse Beaulieu.
Saint-Damien's first settler had arrived in 1824, its first church was built in
1867, and the village received the visit of Monsignor Bourget the following
year.[17] This story meshed perfectly with the one told by Eulalie Riopel. Saint
Damien's original church was demolished in 1960 to make way for a new one.

The two southern towns—Saint-Côme Linière and Saint-Damien-de-
Buckland—were equally tranquil, but further apart from each other. They
seemed to be connected more to larger nearby communities, through the
major autoroute, than they were to each other. No feasts, no pilgrims, no surveys. Correspondence with the diocese of Québec revealed that the designation had been made in 1882 (Saint-Damien) and 1888 (Saint-Côme), but no
records remain to confirm the reasons for the choice. The archivist cautioned
that the towns were far apart and the choice was often made by (or in honor
of) the first priest.[18]

But, as far as we know, the patron saints of the northern pair had been chosen by the bishop because they were doctors and the towns were "born" at the same time. Now, however, the saints' doctoring and even their twinliness had waned through time as communication with large centers improved and distances shrank.

St. Cosmas and Damian of Manhattan

At my first visit to Utica and again in 1995, Bill Dischiavo spoke of another feast day founded by devout immigrants at the Church of the Most Precious Blood on Baxter Street in lower Manhattan. My call was directed to George Minisci, a financial analyst who presided over the Santi Cosma e Damiano Society in lower Manhattan from his home in Bayonne, New Jersey.

Just as the Utica feast related to Alberobello, the rite on Baxter Street is intimately connected to another specific place in Italy: San Cosmo Albanese, a town of some seven or eight thousand people near Cosenza, in Calabria. It was the original home of the founding parishioners; George Minisci was born there too. In the Italian town, he told me, the feast for the medical saints is an exuberant three-day event that can attract up to five or six hundred pilgrims. In 1962, at the age of twelve, George came with his parents to America to join a nonagenarian uncle who had emigrated in 1920. George's brother, Pietro, returned to Italy to serve as a priest at the church in San Cosmo Albanese. As a result, George's understanding of the history of this celebration is a family matter.[19]

The Church of the Most Precious Blood is a large, pale, limestone structure, in the heart of Little Italy near Canal Street. Unlike Saint Francis Church in Toronto, the parish was created in 1888 for the express purpose of serving Italian immigrants. The construction was slow and relied on the energy and fund-raising talents of Franciscan friars who took over the task from the Scalabrini Fathers. From 1903, immigrant parishioners from San Cosmo Albanese marked the feasts of Saint George and Saint Francis, but the doctor saints were soon added at the urging of a parishioner named Cosimo Seremba. He gave paintings of the saints to the church, and eventually the parish raised enough money to purchase wooden statues from a Naples supplier. About a meter high, they are similar to those in San Cosmo Albanese. During the feast, funds are collected to send back to the parish in Italy, partly to relieve poverty and partly to demonstrate the success resulting from life in America. George told me that Manhattan donations have been used for a mosaic in the old church, a loudspeaker, and other modernizations. Gifts continue to be sent to Italy. Planning for the annual feast is the task of the Santi Cosma e Damiano Society.

The Church of the Most Precious Blood is rapidly being engulfed by New York's bustling Chinatown, which has completely taken over Canal Street just a few paces south. Most of the Italian immigrants and their descendants moved away from the neighborhood a long time ago. The church calendar marks other feast days of greater significance, socially speaking. As many of the original parishioners came from Naples, it is the National Shrine of San Gennaro (St. Januarius), their municipal patron. His ornate chapel contains a glass-encased statue much larger than those of the santi medici. Back in Naples, the relic of Saint Gennaro's blood is part of an annual ritual.[20] Its liquefaction on his feast of September 19 is considered a good omen; disaster struck on at least five occasions when the blood failed to liquefy. In 2001, eight days after the September 11 attacks on New York and Washington, the liquefaction was deemed of such reassuring importance that it was reported in the *Italy Daily*.[21] The large, noisy, and messy celebrations for San Gennaro on Baxter Street last a full eleven days and have been featured in Hollywood films. They also mean that the fewer devotees of Cosmas and Damian are confronted with a major cleanup operation before they can prepare the more modest celebration of their own. Long ago, the organizers decided to move the feast for the santi medici to the first Sunday in October, where it has remained. The change in date also placed some psychological distance from the San Gennaro feast, which some dislike for being more sensational and commercial than spiritual.

The Manhattan celebrations to the santi medici are quiet, almost intimate. No more than a hundred attend a solemn morning mass, followed by an hour or two devoted to socializing in the dimly lit, church basement: a catered meal, raffles, other games, and affectionate speeches. There has never been a parade. George acknowledged that secular entertainment is intended to enhance associations for the children and keep them willing to attend. Now into the third and fourth generations after immigration, most of the Manhattan celebrants come from other parishes within a hundred-mile radius ranging from Connecticut to Pennsylvania. Although they are few in total number, the celebrants arrive in multigenerational groups. Most visit the parish only for the Cosmas and Damian feast. George observes that numbers are dwindling: when a grandparent or great uncle dies, the celebration can lose a dozen or more attendees who were loyal to the event out of respect for their elder. A reason to attend the Manhattan feast day, then, is to honor family by pleasing grandparents.

In October 1996, I attended with my daughter, Jessica. The sermon was delivered by a guest priest from the Arborist tradition, which uses the liturgy of John Chrysostom, another Byzantine saint. The priest represented the Sicilian immigrant community of Maria of Grace, New York City's only churchless parish. His sermon drew heavily on parallels between the two communities: both hailed from Magna Graecia of southern Italy; both were striving to maintain faith through devotion to family and tradition. Referring often to Cosmas and Damian as a touchstone, his disquisition mentioned how their roots could be traced to the writings of Patristic fathers such as Theodoret of Cyr, himself known for his sermons. The priest referred to the santi medici for instructive analogies: families should stick together—like twins; the flock should bear witness to faith—like martyrs; neighbors should always be willing to give help—like doctors who cared without fee. In an aside, he observed dryly how few doctors in New York are willing to help anyone without remuneration. He sought support in a community of people who would help a sister-parish because of shared geographic origins and similarly "eastern" patron saints. The congregation was politely quiet, but children fidgeted, and his erudite appeal drifted into the ether.

George's blond, American-born wife is of Ukrainian origin. She and their children attend the feast day every year out of respect for George's family, but she doubts the value of the festival and she predicts that it will not survive. I returned with just a few questionnaires completed. Several members of the Santi Cosma e Damiano Society urged me to visit Howard Beach on Long Island where another feast-day celebration takes place in late August each year.

Cosmas and Damian of Howard Beach

I was beginning to get discouraged. This shapeless project was turning into a painfully awkward, interminable unraveling. Never at ease in telephoning strangers and even less inclined to probe into private forms of devotion, I thought about giving up. Several colleagues pronounced the project inappropriate: it was neither history nor was it medicine; for them, it was not interesting. A few said that, since I was not a sociologist, I shouldn't be wandering in this area and should just go back to reading bone marrows. When another university with a mixed team of sociologists, historians, and anthropologists extended an invitation, I chose to speak about the saints, hoping for some guidance. They were polite but looked bored. One colleague wondered, "Why are you doing this?" I asked for clarification; he replied that the project had little to do with medical history. My answer sounded weak, but it was the truth: "I want to know why these ancient doctors are still being venerated here and now." A former student of mine, who had moved on to graduate studies at that university, revealed that after I left, the professors were more explicitly dismissive; they did not realize his connection to me. Again, credentialism was the issue; the work of sociologists and anthropologists should be read and used only by their professional kin. But I appreciated the feedback.

The negativism of these colleagues contrasted sharply with the eagerness that I found in each community and in casual conversations. At the urging of friends, I put together a story about my experiences with Saint Marguerite d'Youville (I think they'd grown tired of hearing it). *Saturday Night Magazine* accepted it from their "slush pile," creating a little splash of national television and radio appearances that testified to lively interest in the country at large and culminated in two media prizes. Granted the general public was not a peer-review committee, but this attention helped a lot. The wide variety of practices and origins of the devotions to the medical saints deepened and sustained my curiosity. Also, a mild sense of urgency surrounded the gathering of personal recollections of feast-day founders—memories that might soon be irretrievable. The loving enthusiasm that they attached to these ancient doctor saints was fascinating. I suppose that is one reason why I did not give up.

The other reason that I kept going was my friend Bert Hansen, who works at Baruch College of the City University of New York. With Terrie Romano, he was among the few medical historians in my sphere who seemed to like the project. Having begun academic life as a medievalist, Bert was now writing what would become a brilliant, prize-winning history of popular attitudes to medical progress, relying on unconventional sources in mass media, such as comic books, newspaper caricatures, and magazine photographs. He saw the saints' veneration as a manifestation of popular culture that, like his comic books, could have something to say about attitudes to illness, recovery, and health care. Generous and thoughtful, with a big warm smile and a whacky sense of humor, Bert regularly offered a place to stay—and with his deep knowledge of the city's history he was ready for advice about neighborhoods, including Howard Beach, Long Island.

Nevertheless, almost two years passed before I found the courage to telephone all the Catholic churches in Howard Beach, looking for the one that might be home to the santi medici. It was not difficult to find, and once again the reception was warm and open.

A modest suburb of three thousand families, Howard Beach nestles beside JFK Airport. Dozens of times in any hour, a jumbo jet passes low on takeoff or landing. Mafia bosses had made their homes there, and in 1986 racially motivated beatings resulted in a death that drew national attention. Father Francis J. Evans served as parish priest at Our Lady of Grace Church, Howard Beach, for nearly thirty years until his death in 1999.[22] I was fortunate to talk to him in 1998.

Born in the United States of Welsh descent, Father Evans came to Our Lady of Grace Parish in 1972. When asked how the feast-day celebration began, he replied, "Well, I have to admit it was my fault." Shortly after his arrival, an elderly Italian woman stopped him on the street, pointed to his collar, and said: "You priest. Where church?"

This brief encounter exerted a profound effect on Father Evans. He realized that the people had no idea where their church was, and that the spiritual community lacked a center. In an effort to raise interest, he tried to establish a collaboration with the neighboring parish of St. Helen's and was looking for an appropriate saint to honor as a draw for spiritual socializing. Because the two parishes were to be informally "twinned" and many of his parishioners came from Barí, in Puglia, Italy, he welcomed the idea of commemorating the twin saints with an Italian festival, involving a special mass and a socializing. The first event was held on Labor Day weekend 1977, and ten thousand people attended. Father Evans was pleased.

Originally a pretext for people from two parishes to come together around their religion, the celebration's purpose has changed over the years. The life-sized polychrome statues (without beards) were the gift of a parishioner who was deeply devoted to the saints. They were carved in Orvieto, Italy, and transported to Howard Beach, where special cloth garments were made by "a lady of the parish." The companion parish "pulled out" around 1990; Father Evans did not know why. The feast of the twin saints remained solely with the now-singleton church of Our Lady of Grace. But as the twin aspect faded, the medical aspects grew. The celebrants found new purpose in supporting health-care provision. Father Evans had not foreseen this change. He attributed it to a special society founded by the men of the parish, including the donor of the statues.

The International Society of Santi Cosma e Damiano is a nonprofit organization, "founded in 1990," says its brochure, "to continue the works" of the saints "in the health-care field" and to "inform people" of their deeds. The celebration now lasts an entire week in late August rather than on the actual feast day in order to enhance attendance. In addition, to the traditional masses, procession, and music, the events have an unabashedly carnival atmosphere that can attract up to seven thousand people, including "busloads" of regulars from New Jersey. Outdoor vendors rent space for tents, booths, and carnival rides. The proceeds from nightly entertainment and the booths go to support the parochial school adjacent to the church and its yard, while all other funds from the raffles, ticket sales, and gifts are collected for the health-care projects.

This veneration of Cosmas and Damian at Howard Beach strongly identifies with modern medicine. In the years since 1991 gifts of ten thousand dollars or more have been sent to Ronald McDonald House, the Children's Make-a-Wish Foundation, St. Jude Children's Hospital in Memphis, Tennessee, and an adult recovery unit for heart surgery patients at the Roslyn clinic. More recently its largesse has focused on research for autism and juvenile diabetes. Some charities receive donations annually, and the current cumulative total is about $750,000. The society also sponsors a golf outing in May and an annual dinner dance in April with a live band. The lavish printed program for the dinner is complete with thank-you letters from the beneficiaries and images of the saints on the upper corner of every page, including the advertising.

The devoted parishioner of whom Father Evans spoke is Joseph DeCandia. Born to a farming family in Molfetta, Barí, in 1935, he had become a restaurateur and expert pizza maker. Proud of his modest beginnings, his family, and his accomplishments, Joe told his story in the 1998 dinner dance program. Confirming what Father Evans had said, illness interfered with Joe's schooling; his mother "prayed to the saints" and her prayers "worked." Long devoted to Cosmas and Damian, whom he called "his guys," Joe vowed that "if he could get to America, he would let people know about them."[23] He arrived in New York in 1955 with no English. Two years later, he met and married Clara. Gradually, he worked his way up to owning the pizzeria that he had once served as an employee. His expanded operations include a clam bar, a waterside restaurant, and catering service. In 1976 Joe was struck by a car but escaped with minor injuries. He was convinced that the saints saved his life.

Shortly after this accident, Father Evans approached Joe about starting the joint feast-day celebration with the other parish; the statues of the ancient twin doctors arrived soon after. Father Evans was attracted to the twin angle to join two churches; but Joe was keeping a promise. Virtually everyone in Howard Beach recognized Joe as the driving force behind the selection of Cosmas and Damian as the patrons. "He loves those guys!" people say.

Father Evans asked the men of the International Cosmas and Damian Society to circulate my survey at the next feast-day event without my having to travel to Howard Beach. But I promised that I would attend as soon as I could. A clutch of completed questionnaires came by mail in the fall of 1998 reflecting similar patterns to the replies from Utica, Toronto, and Manhattan.

I learned much more by going to Howard Beach in late August 1999 (Figure 3.3). Sadly Father Evans had died and I never met him in person. My husband David came along on the first day and we sampled the good food at the outdoor booths. We spoke with Joe, who was busy making pizza but made time to chat and welcome us. On the second day, I went alone for the services and the procession and to ask questions.

The simple mass took place on Sunday at the end of the celebration week. It was marked by spectacular music—a special song composed for the saints, and a solo of *Ave Maria* sung in the amazing tenor voice of Dan Tomaselli, the music director. Following the service, the members of the International Society display their devotion decked out in tuxedos and black tie. Much admired and photographed by their womenfolk, who form the Ladies Auxiliary, the men assemble to carry the heavy statues through the streets. A priest, "Father Joe," comes from Italy for the celebration every year; he says a special blessing and doves are released.

A significant part of this feast is the procession. No carts or wheels alleviate the burden for the men of Howard Beach as they convey the statues through the community. In a display of devotion (and Catholic manhood[24]), the handsomely dressed "carries," as they are called, hoist the heavy statues on their shoulders—mortification of the muscle. They stride ever so slowly around two or three large blocks, able to manage only a few yards at a time. Working in shifts, they trade places at frequent stops when the statues are set down. Lifting the saints again requires special coordination. During the pauses, the priest bestows blessings, a band plays, and people come out of their homes to visit in the streets and watch the parade pass by. Some observers step forward to pin money to the cloth robes of the saints. Minor deviations from the trajectory bring the statues to visit the sick who are wheeled outside to greet them. About once every minute, a jet departing JFK soars low overhead, but no one seems to mind or notice.

As in Toronto, police stop traffic and an ambulance is at the ready with cool drinks and first aid. Finally the saints are returned to the grounds behind the school. Joe DeCandia's son, Joe junior, retrieves medals that the men had removed from their own necks to place on the statues, while they paid their muscular homage. The local priest, together with Father Joe and Joe senior, then help with the raffle and other entertainment, music, and dancing that will last well into the night. Vendors sell pizza, focaccia, and pastries.

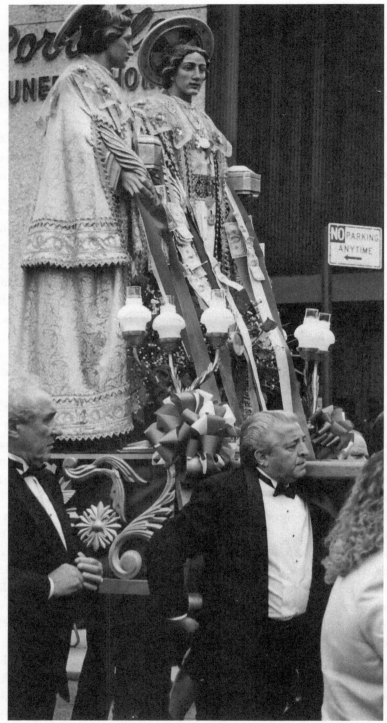

FIGURE 3.3 Joe DeCandia carrying his saints, Howard Beach, NY, 1999.

What had caused the decided shift to supporting health care in 1990? Explanations came from Joe's wife, Clara, and Dan Tomaselli, the music master who also served as special events coordinator. For a long time, Clara and Joe had a pair of statues of the saints in their home and another in their restaurant. One day, Clara was dusting the statues and noticed something odd: their wrists were cracked and oozing, as if they were bleeding. Upset, even frightened, she showed Joe. What did it mean? Together they decided that the saints were trying to communicate with them, that they were sending a message. "They were sad and wanted us to do something."[25] The International Society was the result; it would help the saintly doctors by continuing their work on earth. Joe DeCandia died in 2002, but his son carries on the tradition.[26]

Italian origins and twinliness led to the selection of Cosmas and Damian in Howard Beach; their doctoring provides a reason for social cohesion and the pursuit of good works.

Meanwhile, Back in Toronto

As often as possible, I visited the feast in Toronto. Each time, I would bring along my "survey instrument," but I grew tired of walking up to strangers and interrogating them. By 1998, I settled in to watch, hoping Franca would forgive me. Changes to the pattern of the celebration emerged over the years. It grew to a Triduum—three days of prayer and masses, including an evening ceremony. Saint Michael the Archangel joined the medical saints; his white statue is now carried in the procession too. More recently, the celebrants began to include the popular Italian priest and stigmatic, Padre Pio, who was beatified in 1999 and canonized in 2002. The effigies of the santi medici are sometimes brought outside before the Sunday mass where they wait at the bottom of the steps for the procession to begin. Worshippers leave gifts, or touch the wooden saints' sandaled feet to ask for a blessing as they enter the church.

In 1998, September 27 fell on a Sunday. Two medical students, Julia Cataudella and Ian Billingsley, had been attending a weekend conference in medicine. I offered them a ride back to Kingston, provided that they would wait for me to visit the feast. Julia is a devout Catholic of Italian origin; she was headed for family medicine. Ian had no connection to Italy or Catholicism and was aiming at a future in cardiac surgery, although we had been pushing him to consider internal medicine instead; he seemed too thoughtful for surgery. Ian was amazed at the size of the crowd come to honor a pair of saints of whom he'd never heard.

While we waited and watched, Julia and Ian seemed a tad bored, so I asked if they would like to talk to some pilgrims. I tried to make it clear that they didn't have to—I even told them about my own qualms. True, they may have felt obliged, but each took a bundle of survey instruments and plunged in with admirable fearlessness. Their contributions were profound, not only in the number of forms they completed, but also for what they demonstrated about the research. The people loved talking to the young future doctors. Hearing Julia's Toronto Italian, they lined up to meet her and tell their stories, and soon "la bella dottoressa" was surrounded by more willing candidates than she could interview. Ian found someone who had been operated on by his hero, Dr. Tyrone David, a famous heart surgeon in Toronto. But to his amazement, this man claimed that his heart problem had been cured not by the talented surgeon but by the intercession of Cosmas and Damian. We stayed a long time. Ian took pictures. On the three-hour drive back to Kingston, they chattered about the experience and teased me about my inhibitions.

Ian and Julia showed me that I was getting in the way of my own project— either by being an older woman, a non-Italian, or visibly ill-at-ease, I was putting off the pilgrims. Even if I mustered courage to talk to them, I could not be sure that they would provide honest answers. The idea of research assistants had never struck me as useful because I always preferred to do the digging myself, partly for the sheer joy of archival work and partly for putting myself in the way of noticing connections that might escape a student. But these two students were better at the work than I was.

Cosmas and Damian of Cambridge, Massachusetts

By the late 1990s, we had the Internet and e-mail. Ever vigilant for old comic books and caricatures, Bert began his days with a quick search on eBay, and he passed along links to objects for sale about the medical twins, including paintings, postcards, medals, mugs, and even relics. I was resisting temptation nicely. But then Bert stumbled on www.cosmas-and-damian.org, complete with music. It was May 2001.

An e-mail message sent to the "contact us" button resulted in an almost instantaneous reply from Anthony Leccese, whose warmth and enthusiasm speaks for itself.

Fri, 11 May 2001 22:46:00-0400
    Dear Jackie

I'm delighted to hear from you!

Please call me.

781-XXX-XXXX, I have lots to share with you.

I will also put you in touch with others.

This year is going to be BIG for us. We even have Al Martino for entertainment! Most important to us is our tradition of celebrating our feast day, so you'll find that we are still a very traditional feast with few changes to the way our founders intended the feast to be celebrated. We have great faith in our Saints, and truly believe that these twins heal!

You'll also find that ours is one of the few festivals that is ethnic, but still growing. The organization has many young and old members.

Our, "Old Neighborhood" is diminishing, but the feel of the old days is still present. Many families are still there.

I would really like to talk to you. Please call on a weeknight after 8PM (I have kids). I will not be available on Wednesday the 16th.

I look forward to hearing from you, and naturally would love to have you visit us during the feast.

There is another parish of Saints Cosmas & Damian in Washington state. Have you seen it?

Who could resist? I called and was given a summary of the history of the "Italian Festival of the Healing Saints Cosmas and Damian." Later, I also spoke with Sal DiDomenico, who was organizing the events for that year. His genius for organization was apparent, a talent that surely contributed to his election to the Massachusetts senate in 2010.

Unlike the other sites of veneration, this one in Cambridge was not associated with a particular church. Rather it is the product of an Italian-American society dating back to 1926. The founders were immigrants from Gaeta, Italy, where the twin doctors were patron saints. They worked mostly in the meatpacking industry, as the website explains. Men and women had formed separate organizations in honor of the saints, and a set of statues was ordered from Italy. When the statues arrived, a rift arose from confusion about how they should be carried into the local church, facing forward or backward. They were carried facing forward, which was deemed the "wrong way." The society could thus not remove them and the newly planned tradition was thwarted. As a result, the society henceforth carried out its veneration and its feast independent of the parish, although the rift was healed long ago and religious services are now involved.

In 1948 a piece of land on Porter Street became the "chapel" home for new statues that had belonged to a parish family for its private devotions. Other images and statues of the saints have been gathered—sometimes rescued—and are housed there. Each year in mid-September, a two-day event involves a special healing service, candlelight and daytime processions, entertainment, music, good food, and games for children. In 1988 the community was invited to recreate its festival on the Mall in Washington. By 2001 it was celebrating its 76th anniversary. Its mission is to foster Italian heritage and devotion to its patrons; charitable giving is focused on disadvantaged children. The Washington church of Saints Cosmas and Damian, mentioned by Anthony, had a website with an events calendar that featured no special ceremony on the feast day. It was almost a relief; I had to start setting limits.

Remembering her great success in Toronto, I prevailed upon Julia to go to Cambridge as my research assistant. She had graduated the previous May and was now in the family medicine program at the University of Toronto; she was also engaged to be married, and the ceremony would take place at the Vatican. But she kindly agreed to the task and the organizers at Cambridge treated her like an honored guest. Julia took many pictures and prepared copious notes in the form of a diary. I met with her a few weeks later to go over the findings. She had been included in all the main events and invited to meals *en famille*. She'd even been persuaded to don a chiton (or toga) to participate in the Greek-themed dinner dance. The mayor of Gaeta, Italy, Silvio d'Amante, had been in attendance with his daughter, Chiara, and they invited Julia to visit their feast back home. Clearly this site too—like Toronto, Utica, Howard Beach, and Manhattan—had a link to a specific place in Italy.

Julia had some trouble getting started, but the mayor of Gaeta mentioned her in his remarks to the crowd. She wrote in her diary "[He] focused attention on me! Introduced me, who and where I'm from, described what I am studying—the feast, the miracles, as an MD—spoke of the importance of combination of faith and reason, that faith is also necessary (with medicine) for healing and that sometimes faith plays a greater role than science. This kind and sincere introduction was *very* helpful to me . . . His public support was a blessing." Soon people began lining up to talk to her. Later, one of the organizers told her that "they weren't exactly sure what were the intentions of the work and they had been put off by the word "cult," in my original letter. She confessed her "concern about perceived intrusiveness, but they encouraged [her] to feel free to *be more aggressive*."

While most of the celebrants had roots in Italy, Julia was surprised to meet three women originally from Haiti who lived in Cambridge. She wrote "The meeting with the women from Haiti was striking . . . they said that they 'felt at home' and referred to C and D as 'their saints' and described practices at home involving statues, draping money, and bringing food for the people. It astounded me, as this describes a festival of veneration of C and D arisen in a totally different culture and relatively isolated geographic location."

Results of the Surveys of Pilgrims at Cosmas and Damian Feast Days

In the years of these surveys, 238 forms were completed. The pilgrims ranged in age from under twenty (3) to over eighty (6). Most of the respondents were female, between 63 and 75 percent, with the exception of Howard Beach, where *all* the written responses came from women over forty years of age who had been involved for many years. Important as that celebration is for the men, I suspect that all the questionnaires had been handed to the Ladies Auxiliary. The gender imbalance may have skewed the other survey results coming from that site (Table 1).

This preponderance of women in the surveys reflects several factors. First, it bespeaks a greater number of women attending the feasts, an observation compatible with findings from other studies of Catholic communities.[27] Second, it proclaims their greater willingness to chat and my greater comfort in talking to them; however, my own influence was only partial, since Father Evans had distributed the forms in Howard Beach.

The majority of respondents or their families originated in Italy, but the patterns for Manhattan and Howard Beach were the most circumscribed (Table 1). Almost all those in Manhattan had roots in Calabria near San Cosmo Albanese, and they lived within a one-hundred-mile radius of New York City in New Jersey, Connecticut, Pennsylvania, and Staten Island. Those in Howard Beach lived even closer to their church, most being parishioners; they too had Italian origins, but their families had come from towns such as Genoa and Palermo; one respondent was of Hungarian descent, and two did not answer the question.

In Toronto, the majority came from Italy, especially the south: 38.2 percent from Calabria, 18 percent from Bari, 12 percent from Molise. But some came from Italian sites further north, such as Tuscany, Venice, and Rome. One young woman was Mexican with an Italo-Canadian husband. Another woman was fifty years old and came from Peru. The Toronto pilgrims were

exclusively from the city itself or near its suburbs, such as Downsview, Wood-
bridge, Maple, Scarborough, and Mississauga (Table 1).

In Utica, again the majority hailed from Italy, especially the 24 percent
who cited origins in Puglia where Alberobello is situated. Another 25 percent
came from Calabria (nearly half of whom live now in Canada), but other Italian regions, from Sicily to Venezia, were also represented. Compared to the
other sites of celebration and despite its typically Italian appearance, the Utica
feast seemed less attached to Italian roots. Four people were of Polish origin,
two of Irish, one of Lebanese, one of German-English, and nine admitted to
having "American" roots only. More than 30 percent had traveled from Canadian cities, up to six hours away, such as Kitchener, Niagara Falls, Guelph,
Mississauga, Hamilton, Welland, Saint Catharines, and Toronto. A few came
from New York City. Most of the rest lived within a one- or two-hour radius
in New York State (Table 1).

A few Utica pilgrims are relative newcomers to the feast, but the majority
(80 percent) of those interviewed attend every year. Some seek out friends
whom they met at earlier feasts—people they never see except at the Utica
celebration. I asked the Canadian pilgrims why they do not celebrate in
Toronto. Like the widow whom I met on my first visit, they respond that the
Utica festival is older, bigger, and more authentic, partly because it demands a
greater financial and physical sacrifice. They reminded me of Bill Dischiavo's
observation, "the journey is part of the prayer."

In Cambridge, in addition to the three women of Haitian origin, Julia
found several with mixed ancestry that did not include Italy: five with some
Portuguese background, another five with some Irish, two with Lithuanian,
and one French Canadian. Again the majority were local, but several had
come from the New York City area, one had come from Maine, and another
from Florida—and both those long-distance travelers had been to the feast
more than ten times.

These results support the idea of diffusion, as immigrants brought their
beloved patrons with them to the new world. But at least two of the celebrations, Toronto and Howard Beach, were established many years after the immigration, and factors other than newcomers' longing for the comfort of
home must have been involved (Table 1). Michael P. Carroll noticed the same
pattern elsewhere in his studies of Catholic cults.[28]

The responses to the questions that were designed to help my interpretation were similar in the four centers (Table 2). The saints' medical identity is
more important to pilgrims than their status as twins, although both attributes were recognized. When asked if it was important that the saints were

twins, nearly 70 percent of pilgrims in Toronto and 40 percent or more in Utica, Manhattan, and Cambridge said "yes." Some people supplied personal information to demonstrate that significance: they were twins themselves, or parents of twins, or had twins in their families. When asked if it was important that the saints are doctors, nearly 80 percent of pilgrims in Toronto and a majority elsewhere, except in Howard Beach, responded "yes." Some thought I was mad to ask the question. "Of course, the saints are doctors!" they said. "Good ones too!" Americans often told me jokingly that these saintly medics charge no fees—a good reason to venerate them. This monetary aspect was never cited in Canada. A pilgrim in Cambridge recalled that she once knew a generous Portuguese doctor who treated people without charging fees, just like the saints, but he was now dead. "No doctors heal people for free now," she said.

Tradition and a particular fondness for the saints were the two most frequently cited reasons for attending the feast (Table 3). A striking majority of all pilgrims cited "tradition," especially those in places that strongly identified with particular origins in Italy, such as Cambridge, Utica, and Manhattan. For example, tradition was endorsed strongly by 85 percent of the attendees of the Manhattan celebration, which had been started and maintained by immigrants from San Cosmo Albanese. George Minisci himself told me that was why he had volunteered to organize the event.

An interesting variation on these replies was traditional allegiance to the North American feasts. The Utica and Cambridge celebrations themselves are so old that for these pilgrims "tradition" implied loyalty to the local events in the New World as much as to any ties to Italy: it was chosen by 83 percent of the eighteen people in Utica who did not claim Italian background. In fact, the feast in Cambridge is so tightly associated with Gaeta that one woman of Italian origin whose roots were elsewhere confided that she felt somewhat like an outsider. Nevertheless, she had attended the feast nearly a dozen times and on the occasion that she was interviewed, she had brought along a librarian friend who was both Jewish and Irish and who shared her interests in spirituality and culture.

Almost as important as tradition was a special "fondness" for the medical saints. Overall more than half selected this option as a reason for attending. A handful qualified that response by saying that they were devoted to all saints, but most of these responders knew some stories about Cosmas and Damian—their twinliness, their medicine, their generosity, their martyrdom, and their miracles. Of those who identified fondness for the saints as a reason for attending, 8 percent claimed it was important that they were doctors; in

Toronto that figure climbed to 94 percent while 70 percent of the same group emphasized their twinliness.

Only a few spontaneously admitted that they were seeking specific healings because of illness in themselves or a family member. Sometimes they volunteered this information in response to the question about miracles. In other words, they were hoping for miracles and consulting the saints as doctors.

In exploring the relationship of the North American celebrations in my study to those in Italy and to each other, I asked if pilgrims had attended feasts elsewhere (Table 4). Many had participated in celebrations other than the one where I met them. Sometimes they named events in honor of different saints, but most reported celebrations involving the santi medici elsewhere. In Toronto, twenty people had attended feasts in Italy: four specified Riace or Calabria, three Barí, another three Isernia, but ten offered no precisions. An almost equal number had been to the feast in Utica, and another eleven went to feasts "in the United States," without specifying where.

In Utica, eleven of the eighteen people who had also been to celebrations in Italy live in Canada (Toronto or Kitchener). The other seven live in Utica; five of them had attended original feasts in Barí province at either Alberobello or Bitonto. In Manhattan, a few people had attended the feast in Howard Beach, and four had been to another event in Clifton, New Jersey. Of the eight who had attended the Toronto feast, most lived in that city and only two lived in Utica. Five of the twelve who had been to other American feasts indicated the Utica chapel on Kossuth Avenue as a separate celebration; the remainder mentioned celebrations in Buffalo, Albany, and Endicott.

In Manhattan, a sizeable proportion had been to Italy; only seven of the fifteen specified a town and, for all seven, it was San Cosmo Albanese. Four people, three of whom lived in New Jersey, had attended a feast in that state; one specified Clifton.

In Cambridge, Julia found that eleven people had also been to feasts in Italy at Gaeta, Matera, and Barí; seven had been to Utica. Seven others spoke of their nostalgia for a feast to the santi medici in the Bronx that had ended with the death of an old woman, *la vechietta*, who had been the driving force behind it. Three of these people had traveled to Cambridge from the Bronx because they could no longer attend the feast at home and thought it was important to maintain the devotion. They expressed the wish that it be revived.

About half the pilgrims in both Toronto and Utica said they knew of miracles; some qualified their answers by adding that they had heard of them, believed in them, or were "still waiting" (Table 5). This response rate was surprisingly high in my estimation, and all the more so because few pilgrims claimed that they were attending with healing in mind. Some provided first-hand accounts.

The miracles described by pilgrims are summarized in Table 6. Occasionally, two people would report on the same healing from long ago—a story that had become folk legend. The best example of this is the tale of a Gaeta fisherman, told with variations by several pilgrims. He had been diagnosed with cancer and was advised to put his affairs in order. He went down to the beach to contemplate his gloomy situation. Two men walking along the shore approached him; they instructed him to offer certain prayers and promised that he would be healed. He went out in his boat to pray and recovered completely.

A similar story that took place in the New World was also known to several people. A builder had a urinary problem requiring a catheter, which mortified him. (Some versions contended that the urinary problem was cancer of the kidney.) "Two strangers" told him to return to his doctor because he did not need the catheter. He never knew who these two men were, but he followed their advice and they turned out to be right. The catheter was removed and he recovered. Years later, when he entered the Cambridge chapel to do some repairs, he fell on his knees sobbing and had to be carried out by the perplexed attendants. On first seeing the statues, the builder finally recognized his two strangers as Saints Cosmas and Damian. He did the repairs for free and attends the feast every year.

Most often, however, individuals described cures that had happened to themselves or to close family members, sometimes twins. The illnesses cured were skewed toward life-threatening conditions, such as cancer, heart disease, and severe infections. Accidents and orthopedic interventions were also frequent. Two dealt with threatened blindness. Almost all were healings from physical illness—and they often took place in hospitals. None of the miracles occurred in people who refused to see ordinary doctors. Rather, the saints seemed to provide additional support for contemporary medicine and surgery, which included such drastic interventions as radiotherapy, chemotherapy, electronic cardioversion, and open-heart or orthopedic operations. In one tale, told in Cambridge, doctors misdiagnosed appendicitis and when their patient developed a perforation and peritonitis, they deemed him too frail for an operation; however, he and his wife prayed to the saints and credited them with changing the doctors' minds. Then, after the successful operation, the saints surprised the doctors once more with the man's rapid and complete healing.

Again, like the ancient temple cures of incubation, dreams or visions frequently figured in these stories. The saints would appear the night before an operation, making the surgery unnecessary, or actually performing it, or more often simply reassuring the anxious patient that it was the right thing to do. In these visions they were not always recognized as the medical saints until later, as happened for the builder, above. Sometimes they did odd things: one old woman with breast cancer dreamt that the saints struck her breast with a spear and her tumor resolved without surgery.

Each story had its own dramatic twist. A woman had bought a windshield sticker of the medical twins to place in her father's car as a reminder not to swear so much; it was even beginning to work. Soon after, the father was in a dreadful car accident: the vehicle rolled over and hit three trees; yet he emerged without a scratch. During the crash, he had a vision of what he called, "the two Saint Anthonys." That same night his daughter started awake at 3:35 a.m.—the exact moment of the accident—aroused by Cosmas and Damian, she thinks. Both she and her father are convinced that the saints saved his life.

Some families experienced several miracles, perhaps because they were in the habit of appealing to the santi medici in all their times of woe. A young woman and her husband told me the story of her great uncle: seventy years earlier, he had hitchhiked to the Utica feast to pray for his son, Nick, who according to his doctors was dying of rheumatic fever. Nick survived and grew to be a father himself; he was the woman's uncle. Many years later, her cousin, Nick's seventeen-year-old son, suffered a head injury while playing football and slipped into unconsciousness. The lad's grandmother (wife of the hitchhiker) took up a collection to buy statues of the saints, which she placed by his bed. After a month in a coma, he woke up with no sequelae. Forty years later, Nick's sportive son still has the statues, prays by them every night, and comes annually to the feast, where he and his cousin corroborated the tale.

Similarly, some people credited all their personal recoveries to the saints. Sixty-year-old Elvira from the Bronx told Julia how she had nearly died at the delivery of her daughter thirty-one years earlier. The doctors had planned a Cesarean section, but, due to some medical error, she went into a long and difficult labor and bled. Her mother prayed to the saints, and the local *vechietta* predicted her recovery. During her labor she had a vision of two statues. Three days later, surgery was performed but no abnormalities were found. The doctors, she said, were amazed. Elvira recovered and her child was healthy. Years later in 1995, Elvira was in renal failure and on the verge of dialysis; she came to the Cambridge feast and was overcome with illness at the hotel. One of her daughters went for a doctor, the other brought her a prayer card of

Cosmas and Damian. She prayed to the saints, recovered completely, and did not need dialysis.

Most of these stories concluded with gestures of thanksgiving: a votive offering, such as donation of a "silver arm," or the act of returning to the feast every year—the sacrifice of a pilgrimage. Julia heard of one woman who participated in the procession every year, barefoot, kneeling frequently, and sometimes, people told her, licking the ground.

A few people, especially those in Utica, found miracles in the blessings of their lives: their children, their health, and their freedom. Two described the feast-day event as a miracle because the devotion of the crowd inspires them. One mother saw her son's safe return from Vietnam as a miracle. But the vast majority in all sites construed miracles as physical healing.

From these stories about illness experiences with happy outcomes, several things become clear. First, miracles or acts of grace are largely equated with physical healing and scarcely anything else. Second, almost all the stories of healing involved the care of regular physicians *as well as* an appeal to the saints. Third, incubation may have moved from the temple to the hospital, but it still provides a dominant structure to the healing experience: a striking number of people in all places described visions or dreams of the two saints as part of their recovery stories.

In short, for the religious, it seems, you can scarcely have a miracle without having illness. And most of these miracles happen under medical supervision in ordinary hospitals, but the saints get the credit, not the doctors. Do the health-care providers realize? Probably not. Furthermore, these responses tended to endorse the sociological interpretation that would have the saints filling specific health-care functions, in addition to other spiritual roles.

Cosmas and Damian of Mexico

Of all the colleagues who disapproved of this work, the most disturbing opposition came from my dear friend, Ana Cecilia Rodríguez de Romo. Physician-historian in the faculty of medicine of Mexico City, she too had been in Paris because of her husband's job in the early 1980s, and she too was mother to a young boy. We met in the seminar of our thesis advisor, Mirko Grmek. Sometimes on school holidays, we took turns babysitting our sons so that the other could study. Ana Cecilia's medical expertise was in laboratory medicine and she had written a thesis on the biochemical research of the famous physiologist Claude Bernard. After stints in Fribourg, Switzerland, and in Baltimore, Maryland, she and her neuroscientist husband returned to Mexico. To the immense delight of our advisor, Ana Cecilia and I had both survived professional displacement owing to our family situations, and we had both managed to find medical history jobs in our home countries—jobs that were mirror images of each other. We stayed in touch, visited in our homes, sent copies of our publications, and attended history of medicine meetings together. She took me to Teotihuacán. I took her to Lake Louise. Our sons grew up in parallel—hers became an orthopedic surgeon and mine a physicist. Her father and my mother died in the same year, and much later, within the same week of 2008, we both became grandmothers of little boys who have yet to meet, Rodrigo and Tycho.

By October 1998 Ana Cecilia was doing very well personally and professionally. Petite, beautiful, dark, and very articulate, she was stepping down from the prestigious presidency of the National Society of Medical History in Mexico. The first woman to serve in that capacity, she had reached this pinnacle at a relatively young age. Her presidential address would be given at the annual meeting, and she had invited me and our mutual friend Anne-Marie Moulin. The meeting was held in the marvelous eighteenth-century city of Québetaro, not too far from the artist colony of San Miguel d'Allende. I took along Jessica to complete our gang of four, and we traveled about in Ana Cecilia's blue Volkswagen Beetle.

At the meeting, Ana Cecilia delivered a brilliant address, and Anne-Marie also spoke very well in fluent Spanish. I could not do that, but the audience was kind and relatively accustomed to English. Using an updated version of the paper from Holland, I told them about the Cosmas and Damian work, partly because I wanted to know about the veneration in Mexico, and this seemed the best way to spread the word. No one complained and several people told me of the church and the hospital dedicated to the medical saints in Mexico City.

Perhaps the topic embarrassed Ana Cecilia; she seemed preoccupied by my deviating from our usual subjects. That year, I had finally published my thesis on the invention of the stethoscope, of which she thoroughly approved, happily drawing it to the attention of her colleagues. Pediatrician Max Shein and his psychologist wife Rosita liked that new book especially because I had mentioned the role of music in the inventor's life. With a vast knowledge of medical history, they are experts and collectors of pre-Columbian art and musical instruments. But they also seemed to understand my interest in the saints, and took me to a historic pharmacy in San Miguel.

But Ana Cecilia kept wondering why I was working on saints and religion. I asked what bothered her about it. Her reply was blunt: it is not medicine; it is not scientific; and it is not interesting. She seemed worried that I would lose credibility in our field. After the conference, it was time to relax. Over meals at the outdoor taverna, late-night margaritas, and hanging about in the pool at her splendid country home at Chiconcuac, it was mildly distressing to have to keep justifying the project. I think Anne-Marie was bored.

I pressed Ana Cecilia on her objections. She seemed to have a horror of the church's control over people's lives, as if society had moved beyond all that. Confidence in science was the opposite of religion, which, for her, was superstition, wishful thinking, and irrational. Traditions were quaint, but it was good that the people could now put these primitive beliefs far behind them. There is no need to resurrect them. She understood that I was not advocating religion, but as far as she was concerned, I was going backwards from what we do best, and I was leaving the much more interesting medical science behind.

Ironically, these tense conversations played on a background of the upcoming festivity of Dia de los Muertos, the Mexican celebration of All Saints' Day or Halloween. Adding to the usual vibrant color of the country, market stalls sold tiny sugar skulls, massive paper flowers, and special foods to be taken to the cemeteries for graveside picnics in honor of the dead. Random displays all over the cities featured skeletons in bizarre activities—playing electric guitars, or typing on computers. Even Ana Cecilia had set up a shrine of sweets for her grandmother on a low table in her living room. Jessica was soon to turn fifteen, a coming-of-age moment for girls in Mexico, and she was especially indulged with these "muertos" goodies and other gifts.

Then to our amazement, Ana Cecilia told us that as a child she had attended the Cosmas and Damian church with her grandmother. Nothing is close in Mexico City, but she offered to take us there. It is north and slightly west of center; both the neighborhood and its subway station are called San Cosme. We arrived on a brilliant, sunny morning and passed through a well-groomed courtyard into the ornate church that featured a vast golden reredos surrounding statues of the medical twins. A priest was only too pleased to speak with us in French—literally our *lingua franca*—because he was from France. He seemed to think it was intentional that we had arrived just minutes before the monthly service for healing of the sick, a tradition that had been part of the parish long before he arrived. We found the coincidence lucky, almost too good to be true, and stayed to watch. The small congregation contained a few people with obvious infirmities, but the priest explained that many who attended this mass were praying for someone else. At one point, Ana Cecilia fell on her knees. Jess and I looked at each other, wondering if she was ill or overwhelmed by a flood of memories for her much-loved grandmother, or simply worn out from the exhausting cycle of meetings and visitors.

Not one to hold a grudge, my friend soon forgave me and sent books and articles pertaining to religion and medicine and the founding of hospitals in Mexico.[29] Cosmas and Damian came to Mexico with the Europeans, arriving there a long time before they came to the United States or Canada. For centuries, hospital medicine was the purview of religious people in that country. The Amor de Dios hospital was established in 1539 near the site of the present-day church by the first archbishop, Juan de Zumárraga; Cosmas and Damian were its protectors, their images graced the entrance, and people often referred to it by their names. While some indicate that the hospital was to care for Indians, other sources claimed that it catered more to Spaniards; its main focus was syphilis, hence its nickname "Las Bubas." Another role entailed public health by segregating the sick to protect the healthy invaders. It was not the first hospital in New Spain. Somewhat earlier in 1524, the Spanish conquistador Hernando Cortes had founded what is now called the Jesus Hospital; the remarkable buildings visible there today are from the early seventeenth century. In 1570 another San Cosme y San Damián hospital appeared in Oaxaca, and in 1617 the brothers of John of God founded yet another in the city of Léon, Guanajuato. One of the earliest tourists in Mexico, Father Alonso Ponce, visited dozens of convents over a five-year period in the 1580s, among them the monastery to the medical saints.[30] Physicians, surgeons, barbers, chaplains, and nurses worked within the walls of the Cosmas and Damian hospital according to a strict set of rules. From the outset, the "best doctors" were engaged in this service, such as Christobal Ojeda and Pedro Lopez who had arrived with Cortes; the first surgeons were Diego de Pedraza and Francisco de Soto.

The present church and its cloister date from 1672. Historians emphasize that these institutions began with religious caregivers rather than doctors, and that they were aimed at spiritual as well as physical healing. Cosmas and Damian arrived with, and participated in, European medicine.

The Fourth and Fifth Papers

I could not survey all these places and pilgrims and I did not want to try. Ana Cecilia's negative opinion mattered a lot and forced me to reexamine my motives. She seemed to be the honest friend who would interpret and help reorient my quest. Always looking for advice, I had been submitting papers on

Cosmas and Damian for history of medicine meetings, but my proposal for the 1997 meeting of the American Association for the History of Medicine had been rejected. At the time, I'd assuaged disappointment and responsibility with luck-of-the-draw resignation. But Ana Cecilia's opinion suggested that other researchers in our field probably agreed with her. I also used opportunities to air the work in scholarly centers: an invitation came from Guenter Risse to speak in San Francisco, another from the Wellcome Centre in London, England, and yet another from the New York Academy of Medicine. Most of these distinguished audiences listened politely, but no one had any suggestions as to what to do with the work. Embarked on his monumental history of hospitals, Risse was more sympathetic than many colleagues, and he understood both the fascination and the problems. He repeatedly ran up against the role of religious actors in his study of hospital history; their involvement went far beyond the financial concerns of hospital management to tilt at medical epistemology—the very meaning of illness, disease, treatment, and healing. He agreed that, in a kind of intellectual apartheid, the existing literature in modern medicine did not address these problems.

The most supportive comments came from medievalists who could not study medical history without also studying religion. Thus it was that in November 1999 an e-mail arrived from my Queen's University colleague in history, Monica Sandor, about a conference on "Saints and the Sacred," upcoming at Saint Michael's College, Toronto:

> Date: Mon, 29 Nov 1999 19:30:10 = 0500
> To: duffinj@post.queensu.ca
> From: Monica Sandor sandworm@qsilver.queensu.ca>
> Subject: conference on saints
> Jackie,
> I wondered if you might be interested in this upcoming conference on saints—either to present your stuff on medical miracles and saints (they especially would like people from the sciences to participate!) or to attend, if you are interested enough in the topic. It is not meant to be solely medieval.
> Monica

Bless Monica! This meeting seemed perfect for my needs, and the University of Toronto was my medical alma mater. Moreover, it was a mere three hours down the road—no airplanes involved. I was excited when my paper was accepted, but daunted by the fact that I'd been placed first on the program, forcing me to confront a completely unknown audience. I arrived early to make sure that my slides would work. The organizer, Professor Joseph Goering, also came early to help set up. It quickly emerged that I was one of only a few planning to use slides and, as might have been predicted, I was the only "scientist." Minutes later, a dashing, dark man stalked in, furious that the volumes from last year's meeting had not yet arrived from the printer for their promised distribution. Cursed with a strange blend of Mediterranean passion and Teutonic order, he fumed noisily for a while, stopped, noticed that I was a stranger, and shook my hand with a warm smile. This was Goering's colleague, Francesco Guardiani, an expert in seventeenth-century Italian poetry.

The interdisciplinary group who teach at Saint Michael's College come from history, theology, music, languages, art history, and philosophy. They provoke collaboration across their academic silos with this once-a-year collo-quium around a common theme. I was fortunate that they had chosen saints and that my saints were Torontonians. For the first time ever, the paper went well. Although no one told me what to do with the work, no one told me to stop. At the social gathering in the evening, many people expressed interest and encouragement for the research—with no question of its belonging. I offered my paper for the proceedings; it became my first Cosmas and Damian publication—a decade after the work began. More exciting, even propitious, was the subject of their conference planned for 2001: miracles.

A year later, I returned to Saint Michael's College. This time I knew several people and felt quite at home, although few of the scholars ventured beyond the shoals of the nineteenth century. Having accomplished some of the pil-grim surveys, I summarized the findings so far, featuring the miracles, and re-lated the work to the theories that I'd been toying with for more than a decade. I concluded that, with their significance to Italian immigrants and their sur-prising involvement in health care, the best reason why Cosmas and Damian were now in Toronto was that they filled social and medical functions.

The wide room with a window wall at the back was packed. But for some reason the audience was accidentally distributed in a gender-unequal fash-ion. Women, including a few nuns, sat to my left. Men, most professors, a few clerics, and graduate students, were to my right. Questions were polite and easy, until I recognized a hand at the back right: it belonged to Giulio Silano, professor of Christianity and culture. He challenged the fact that I had accepted the healing stories of pilgrims as "miracles." These healings, he insisted, were lesser events—"acts of grace." A real miracle was something else that had to withstand rigorous, formal scrutiny. In the heat of the mo-ment, I defended myself by saying, "If interview subjects thought fit to use the word 'miracle,' I didn't think it was my place to tell them otherwise." An audible cheer went up from the left side of the room. But Silano had a good point. How did the miracle stories of my pilgrims differ from the official ones found in the Vatican? Did the forms of veneration in North America really resemble those back home? I had been assuming that they were similar, but I had no evidence.

For two reasons, I had to go to Europe: to compare the feast-day events to those back home and to search for the nature of "real" miracles. Now it was time to apply for a grant.

TALKING TO PILGRIMS had provided some surprising evidence in favor of the medical role of Saints Cosmas and Damian in our time. But it had done little to advance one theory over another. Indeed it had raised more questions. If the feasts were strictly imitative of those back home, then the discovery of non-Italians, nonparishioner pilgrims—like the Haitians in Cambridge and the Poles in Utica—needed more explanation than diffusion and genealogy. Perhaps, the forms of veneration had evolved following the initial migration of the santi medici: with exposure to our health-obsessed culture, had their function in North America grown more medical than it was in Europe? And what did that health-care activity, implicit in the many so-called "miracle" stories of my pilgrims, have to do with the official miracles of canonized saints?

4

Chasing Saints in the Old World

*Romantic and historic sites, such as the land of Italy abounds
in, offer the artist a questionable aid to concentration when
they themselves are not the subject of it. They are too rich in
their own life and too charged with their own meanings
merely to help him out with a lame phrase; they draw him
away from his small question to their own greater ones.*
—HENRY JAMES, *The Portrait of a Lady, Author's Preface, 1907*

IN THE EARLY 1980s, French national television aired a program called,
"*La chasse aux trésors.*" A kind of scavenger hunt designed to feature exotic
parts of the world, it starred Philippe de Dieuleveult, a hyperenergetic demi-
god who would jump, ride, run, swim, or fly, at the commands of erudite
competitors from the safety of the Paris studio. Given a few clues, rival teams
would triangulate on the designated *trésor* with history books and travel
guides. "Philippe! Philippe! Come in, Philippe!" they would call into head-
sets to send their errant knight off in another direction. The audience was
led to think that the search against the clock occurred in real time. But full
enjoyment demanded surrender of disbelief. Once, Dieuleveult dove out of a
helicopter into the sea where an underwater camera linked to the television
network just happened to be lurking ready to capture him breaking the surface. He vanished on a dangerous rafting expedition in Zaire in 1985; some
think it was murder. Ever after, my family used "Philippe! Philippe!" as code
for the quixotic, ridiculous, or wild tangents that ricochet off the still facade
of academic composure.

Our search for the medical saints was a little like "*La chasse aux trésors.*"
Armed with a bizarre combination of histories and travel guides, David and
I targeted the sites of feasts that had spawned North American progeny.
Present-day sanctuaries of Cosmas and Damian are unevenly distributed:
intense concentrations in some geographic regions, sparse in others. The

locations seem not to be an accident; however, as many chapels and churches can trace their origins to an early medieval past, the precise reasons and dates of founding are now obscure and almost impossible to uncover. In her work on France, Marie-Louise David-Danel suggested several hypotheses as to why some places venerate the medical saints more than others: transposition on to anterior sites of healing; arrival of their relics; and connection to pre-existing medical activities in the region.[1] Using her extensive repertoires and those of Pierre Julien, I generated a list of sites to visit; it was conditioned by my pilgrim surveys: Alberobello, Gaeta, Riace, and Isernia were high on that list. But we would also stop at lesser feasts and sites that venerated the saints. We could not be at every shrine for the precise feast day, but a month's journey in Italy, during the two weeks leading up to the feast and the two weeks following, might make it possible to find organizers and explore local traditions. We planned to be in Alberobello for the actual feast.

All this reasoning was explained in my grant application to the Hannah Institute for the History of Medicine. It was enormously encouraging to receive peer approval and the timing was perfect as David and I were both on sabbatical leave for the academic year, 2001–2002. Other notions had been too flimsy for mention in the grant application. For example, we would look for the saints near the ancient cities known to have had temples to the twin Dioscuri or to Asklepios, the ancient god of medicine. I had also begun to nurture the idea that the North American feasts were wealthier and more medical than those in Europe and that this scientific emphasis had evolved since the migration of the cults. Consequently, I was expecting to assess the relative splendor of the events and the focus of their philanthropy.

These ideas could be tested only by actually going to the places of veneration. First, however, I wanted the advice of the distinguished historian of pharmacy, Pierre Julien, who seemed to know all about these places already.

Paris

Tall, thin, bespectacled, and soft-spoken, Pierre Julien kindly welcomed me to his elegant apartment between the Pantheon and the Jardin de Luxembourg. I had never seen anything like his fabulous collection. Every wall, every cabinet, every horizontal surface bore something relating to the holy twins. More objects hid in drawers and cabinets: paintings, humble lithographs, icons, prayer cards, bookplates, crockery, medals, fridge magnets, key chains, clothing, calendars, seals of confraternities, and statuettes of multiple sizes and shapes in stone, glass, wood, plaster, plastic, and pastry.

Julien's books and articles were familiar, but he had written about only a minuscule fraction of what he owned and knew. Generous and patient, his face lit with delight, he explained the provenance and charms of favorite objects. Several fat albums contained photographs taken on his journeys to various feast-day celebrations.

Among the ephemera were many duplicates of simple, paper posters announcing "goigs" (celebrations) in honor of the medical saints. This Catalan word, also *gozos* and *goggius*, is derived from Latin "gaudia," and means a poem or song of praise. The posters came from different years and many villages in a circumscribed area of Catalonia surrounding Girona and extending to both sides of the border with France. Known in Spain since the ninth century, it seems that veneration to the "*sants metges*" increased in that region with each passing epidemic.[2] For example, the French border town of Argelès-sur-Mer suffered an outbreak of plague that disappeared on September 27, 1652; the population vowed to make a solemn procession to honor their patrons every year since that time.[3] Pierre Julien's many "goigs" announcements came from villages and towns in the dioceses of Barcelona, Tarragon, and especially Girona. Exhibitions of goigs posters have taken place. Scholars point to their utility in social history, and because they are printed in limited numbers, they have become collectors' items; those in honor of the medical saints represent only a modest fraction of the whole. The veneration in Catalonia seems to still be evolving and growing. For example, just outside Saint Julia de Ramis near Girona is an eleventh-century shrine atop a wooded hill once inhabited by Romans and Visigoths. It receives an annual pilgrimage to the medical saints, but the actual dedication of the sanctuary to the medical saints was established only in 1943, when a new, large parish church to Saint Julia was built along the main road.

Pierre Julien carefully studied the list of places that I planned to visit, approving, warning, and offering names of contacts. One invaluable bit of advice entailed looking for giant posters, an Italian practice to announce times and locations of events in the local *feste*. Photographs of these posters, he said, would save a lot of time later in reconstructing the celebrations. We stayed in touch over the year by letter and telephone. This man was far more obsessed with the saints than I. He thought it was utterly normal that we would do this running around and call it research.

My friends François and Martine Gallouin drove me out to the Cosmas and Damian church at Luzarches, north of Paris near Charles de Gaulle airport. Julien had described its long history as a Christian community since the eighth century and as a site of veneration of the medical saints since at least the twelfth century if not before. Around 1160 the returning crusader, Jean de Beaumont, brought relics—the arms of the santi medici—from Rome to France, placing them in Paris and Luzarches, where the Collégiale Saint Cosme was established.[4] According to a fourteenth-century inventory, one arm was already missing. In 1260 groups of doctors, dentists, and surgeons united in a single Parisian confraternity, the Confrérie Saint Cosme. Loyal members offered gratis services on the first Monday of every month, and they went the twenty-four miles to Luzarches each September 27th in honor of Cosma and Damian.[5] During the atheism of the Revolution, the confraternity was suppressed, the church damaged, and its relics dispersed. But Catholic doctors remained attached to its significance, and devotion was quickly reestablished. In the way that research projects tend to collide with each other, I learned that René Laennec, the boldly Catholic inventor of the stethoscope, had journeyed there as an act of piety and inspiration. The town now has a hospital and a street named for him, and a group called le Cercle Laennec organizes pilgrimages for doctors and pharmacists.[6] In the twentieth century, other relics were transferred to Luzarches, and it became a repository for statues and paintings of the medical saints, including a fine canvas by the neoclassical artist Jules Alexandre Duval-Lecamus.

While in France, we visited old friends and tied up loose ends dangling from the project on the stethoscope. As a result, we found ourselves in Brittany, where Laennec had lived, and where saints, shrines, and healing wells are legion. What I had never before appreciated was how many of these sites also venerate Cosmas and Damian. Wells that had been sacred in the religion of the Celts were simply co-opted by Christians and assigned protector saints to replace their earlier sprites. For example, tiny but ancient chapels to the medical twins can be found at Saint Nic (Finistère), Lusanger (Loire-Atlantique), Naizin (Morbihan), and fountains at Saint Nic and Plomeur (also Finistère). David-Danel documented many Breton sites that possess sculptures and statues, and she wrote admiringly of their distinctive attributes. "Anyone who has trouble understanding how a stature can be both hideous and exquisite needs to go to Brittany." Or, "In deepest Finistère, the sanctuary of Saint-Côme at Saint Nic—with its beautiful, wooden rafters, its Calvary statues gnawed by sea air, and its fountain that flows beneath the feet of the stone saints in the nearby meadow—constitutes an irresistible ensemble of poetry and artistic value."[7]

These observations shook my confidence. With so many different forms and manifestations of devotion to the medical and other saints, how would visiting some shrines in France and Italy explain the current veneration in Canada? I had to keep focused on the threads that led to North America.

Geneva

We rented a Renault Mégane. David would do the driving and I would navigate. We were apprehensive about going back to Italy—we'd been badly robbed there in 1990 and the roads were treacherous. En route, we stopped in Geneva for David to conduct some interviews as part of his own research and to visit with Ann Pollack, our good friend from his diplomatic days in Paris. While waiting, I visited Voltaire's house, the History of Science Museum, and the World Health Organization. Our Mexican friends Max and Rosita Shein were in town; over a delicious Ferney-market lunch provided by Ann, we chattered about the planned journey and I drew courage from their continued approval. We planned to leave Geneva on September 12, 2001. The day before our departure, I stayed home with Ann, who was not feeling well. All our anxieties about Italian travel and the project itself shriveled in significance with the terrifying pall that swept the world on that horrible day. Air travel came to a halt, border crossings ground to a crawl, and no one knew what would happen next. But we were freakishly free to drive from Switzerland into Italy, chasing saints. "Philippe! Philippe!"

Italy

The plan was to travel quickly south to Sicily and slowly work our way back north. But Geneva to Trapani cannot be accomplished overnight. We made Lerici on the first night at the eastern end of the Riviera. The hotel sent us to *Il Pescatore*, a legendary taverna where a multicourse fish meal simply appeared—no menu, just delicious food, all fish—highly recommended. Reliable information about what was happening was hard to come by, and dazed diners swapped stories. A pair of American newlyweds had been airborne at the moment of the terrorist attacks. They learned about the disaster hours later when they landed in Italy, by which time the route home was barred. "Enjoy your honeymoon." We kept going.

Latina

The town of Santi Cosma e Damiano (pop. 6,800) is lost in the dry hills between the sea at Gaeta and the autoroute below Monte Cassino. According to Pierre Julien, it is the only municipality in the world to bear the name of both saints. Thanks to the narrow twisting road, we arrived much later in the afternoon than planned. The church was easy to find, but tragically plain, a postwar reconstruction in concrete. Multiple war memorials explained why, striving not to assign blame in one direction or another; in the lengthy, destructive battle of Monte Cassino in 1944, the hapless town had been on the Gustav Line, so it was right in the way of both the German retreat and the Allied advance.

Short statues of the patron saints had been moved to the center aisle of the church, but nothing seemed to be happening inside or out. Anxious to be in Gaeta itself before dark, we grabbed a coffee and strolled a bit, looking for the giant posters with the schedule of events that Pierre Julien had recommended. Just as we were about to go back to the car, a voice with a startling London accent said, "Don't leave yet. The people just are about to have a little parade. Stay to watch." Silvio was sitting at the café with several other men of a certain age. He had been born in the house across the street—the one with the green door. Now a chef in London, he returned every year for two or three months.

"How long 'till the parade?"

"Any minute now," he said, pointing to the giant poster beside him. It suggested the parade should have been going for half an hour already.

We lingered. Banners were being draped around the church door by a young woman and her children. Two hours later, people were still wandering slowly toward the church, up its steps and into the interior darkness. Silvio shrugged. "They *will* carry the statues around the town and put them back inside the church," he promised. But we didn't wait.

Gaeta (pop. 22,700)

Gaeta is the original home of the founders of the feast-day celebrations in Cambridge, Massachusetts. A walled medieval town occupying a sunny headland, its modern spillover extends around the southern shore of its gulf with palm trees, piazzas, and banks. The narrow older streets admit only motor scooters and laundry. Greco-Roman antiquities attest to its occupation for nearly three millennia. A local cave purports to be the dwelling of the Cyclops. Gaeta, too, suffered grievously in World War II—the citizens were expelled as the Germans made it a garrison.

We raced to the cathedral, but the feast-day celebrations were not immediately obvious; Gaeta's shrine must be off the beaten path. A poster on the door gave us hope but no directions. Julia Cataudella's encounter in Massachusetts was still two weeks off, and we had no insider information. For the discerning tourist, content to ignore the seductive beach, Gaeta's two main attractions are the castle and the Duomo cathedral, with its Sicilian "moorish" influence and late thirteenth-century Paschal candelabrum encrusted with low reliefs. We stopped at another ancient church, Santa Maria Annunziata, where a diminutive nun knew of Gaeta's santi medici. But before she would reveal directions of how to find them, she insisted that we visit the magnificent Renaissance room, called the Capella d'Oro, where Pope Pius IX is said to have deliberated before approving the Bull of papal infallibility.

Even with the nun's directions, the church was difficult to locate; it lay in the more modern section of town. Its approach cut across dark, interior streets, too narrow for a car—and was easy to miss, but shockingly bright and open when found. A wide stairway led up to the door. The pale, blue interior housed a statue of the virgin and small statues of the santi medici. Plans were underway for the feast-day celebrations, but the priest was engaged in an interminable telephone call. Two women assistants who understood my quest had no schedules or information left, last year's being all gone and this year's overdue from the printer. Come back in three days, they said.

It was just as the people in Cambridge, Massachusetts, had said: their American feast was much larger than the one back home.

Sicily

David careened down the autostrada, over bridges and through tunnels, to Reggio di Calabria on the straights of Messina. The following day we crossed to Sicily. In looking for the santi medici, I now could give free rein to the attractive hypothesis that they descended from well-developed pagan cults of the ancients who had occupied the region—cults devoted to healing, or to divine twins. Settled from the eighth to the sixth century BC, Magna Graecia included Sicily and the southern coast of Italy, from Cumae just north of Naples to the region near present-day Taranto in the south. Archeological excavations of these ancient Greek cities display layouts of the principal buildings and temples: many had cults dedicated to the god of medicine, Asklepios, or to the twin Dioscuri, or, like Agrigento's Valley of the Temples, to both.

The Greek influence in southern Italy also persists in language, cultural practices, and religious customs. Long after Magna Graecia fell to Roman rule, eastern traditions remained relatively more resistant, attractive, and accessible in this part of Italy. Later, the orthodox Christian traditions also had a stronger foothold in the south. Byzantine rule persisted even longer in Sicily than it did in Ravenna. Mass was said in Greek until the Arabic conquest in the tenth century. These lingering influences had been part of the sermon delivered by the Arborist priest in Manhattan.

We saw Segesta, Agrigento, and Taormina. It was exciting to find ruins of a temple to Castor and Pollux and another to Asklepios at Agrigento. If the other places had such temples, it was not easily visible to random tourists like us. Shrines to Cosmas and Damian are indeed numerous in the vicinity of these ancient Greek cities—but it is wishful thinking to imagine one could demonstrate that the saints' prominence in Magna Graecia might be owing to these pagan roots. Greek or Roman towns of any respectable size would have had temples to the Dioscuri and Asklepios, and only some of these sites have been identified and excavated so far. Moreover, the identity of each temple was uncertain, established by convention and scholarly argument. Evidence for the veneration of the saints, whether in objects, buildings, or documents, can be extended only as far back as the eleventh century. A gaping hiatus of a millennium could not be ignored. Furthermore, the proximity of pagan temples to Christian shrines for the santi medici need not represent cause and effect—or a continuity. It might be just coincidence.

Equally plausible is the possibility that the saints were brought to Italy during Byzantine rule. Their origin in the east, combined with the gratitude of Emperor Justinian for the cure that he attributed to their intervention, made them famous in Constantinople. Little wonder, then, that they would travel to the far-flung corners of his empire with its citizens. The twin saints are portrayed in the remarkable sixth-century mosaics of Saint Andrea chapel in Ravenna, thought to date from the year 545, long before the arrival of relics.[8] Similarly, they are also prominently depicted, much larger than life, in the astonishing gold mosaics of Monreale south of Palermo, which date from the twelfth and thirteenth centuries.

Sferrocavallo (pop. 5,300)

Ask any cab driver in Palermo for the santi medici and you will be whisked to Sferrocavallo. Literally meaning "iron horse," Sferrocavallo is a quaint fishing village tucked under a towering rock, a short distance west of Palermo. Cosmas and Damian are its patrons. A new monument dedicated to the saints stands in the harbor: Janus-like, the statues face out to the sea and also inland to the town center. The parish church is under the protection of the santi medici, and its elaborate, weeklong celebration, with illuminations, processions, concerts, and miracles, is famous throughout Sicily. The highlight is the Ballo dei santi, a procession going back to the eighteenth century or earlier, during which the devout transport the statues through town on a heavy dais. As soon as the feast is over, preparations begin for the next year. Intricate, lacework arches of lights had already been mounted above several streets, and the multiple events of the feast, both religious and secular, were proclaimed on large posters, plastered on windows and walls, every few feet throughout the village. Anneliese Wittmann studied the Sferrocavallo feast day as an archetypical Sicilian celebration; here the saints may be doctors, but their responsibilities are the safety and success of fishermen.[9]

Naro (pop. 8,700)

Sicilian Naro, just twelve miles from Agrigento, rises out of an arid but fertile plain. Drenched in warm afternoon sunlight, Naro slept as we arrived: shops were closed and the streets empty. We headed for the *chiesa matrice*. A big poster on the door announced the forthcoming feast-day celebrations for the santi medici. I had hoped that this church would be their shrine, but a quick tour around its pastel interior confirmed that it was not. A children's choir was practicing, perhaps for the feast. One singer, called Serena, told me that they were rehearsing for a wedding. The children gathered round and raised their voices now in chatter, happily explaining how to find the Chiesa Sant'Agostino where the santi medici resided. They knew all about the feast day, even though it did not belong to their parish.

The fortified church of Sant'Agostino of Naro and its convent stand on the western edge of town on a hill overlooking the splendid dry valley to the north. Tall, fortress-like, and almost windowless, it has the air of a Saracen castle rather than a church; it was founded in the twelfth century and restored in the eighteenth. Inside, white flowers were tied to the pews and huge bouquets stood at the foot of the chancel. On either side of the altar were graceful, polychrome, wooden statues of Cosma and Damiano, about half of life size, perhaps of seventeenth- or eighteenth-century making (Figure 4.1). A photographer, who was setting up for the wedding, described the feast-day events. The church would be full. There was no procession that he could recall, but sick people came to pray, as did some doctors.

Outside on the church steps, an elegantly dressed crowd had gathered, dwarfed in the shadow of the immense building behind them. A shiny black car pulled into the piazza with what seemed like unnecessary speed, screeching to a stop as far from the church steps as was possible in that empty space. On her father's arm, the diminutive bride floated slowly across the piazza in her billowing white dress, catching the late afternoon sun at just the right angle to generate applause. This is how one marries in

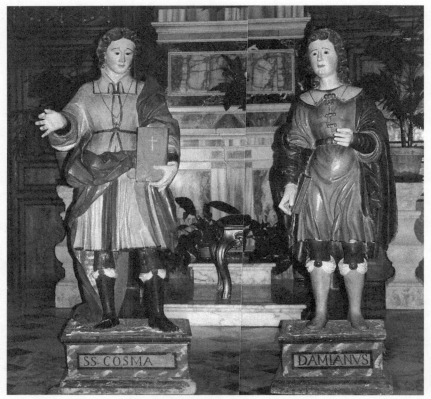

FIGURE 4.1 Statues of the santi medici, Naro, Sicily, 2001.

Naro—a tremendous photo-op prior to consecrating a union under the benign gaze of the santi medici. It turns out this is also how many people marry throughout Italy.

Riace (pop. 1,600)

We took the ferry back to the mainland from Messina—an important site from a medical history perspective. Only four miles wide, the treacherous straight was known to sailors in Homeric antiquity; fearsome monsters clung to the rocky headland of Scylla along the mainland and the whirlpool of Charybdis swallowed sailors whole, sometimes with their ships. In the autumn of 1346, Genoan vessels sailed into the harbor of Messina from the eastern Mediterranean bringing that dreadful pestilence, later called the Black Death. Guide books do not mince words: Messina has been destroyed many times by earthquakes, plagues, and bombs.

We were headed to Riace, on the underside tip of Italy's great toe. Several Torontonian Italians recalled the feast-day celebrations in that town. There seemed to be only one hotel in the vicinity. With a famous festival about to begin, we had called ahead to reserve. The Hotel Federica was new, comfortably simple, and ideally situated on the beach at Riace Marina. But it was virtually empty. The hotel receptionist knew of the *festa*, but she was not expecting pilgrims. She shrugged amiably and said that they would *never* stay in a hotel.

Enchanting Riace village, four miles inland at an altitude of 300 meters, is suspended sling-like across the upper end of a dusty valley strewn with cactuses, olive groves, and sheep. On clear days, the Ionian Sea is visible between the brown hills. Cosmas and Damian have been the town patrons for centuries. Scholars suggest that the santi medici of Riace inherited a peasant celebration that had itself emerged from an ancient rite for rain, and was once the purview of the pagan god, Jove. With roots in antiquity, then, it claims to be the oldest Italian site of veneration to the santi medici. Natives of nearby Stignano contest this story and assert that the Italian veneration of Cosmas and Damian began in their town.

But documents trace these origins only as far back as a convent, founded by Bartholomew Atulino and placed under the protection of the santi medici.[10] The monastery flourished from the sixth to the eleventh century; supposedly it featured a painting of the Redeemer embracing the two saints in a grotto. A lay confraternity was established at Riace in 1637, and relics were donated by the Bishop of Squillace in 1669 and 1671. Under Napoleon, however, the confraternity was suppressed, only to be revived in 1835.[11] The members of the confraternity still look after preparations for the celebrations. A permanent pillar, in colored tiles portraying the saints' lives, marks the narrow road to the sanctuary of the santi medici, about a half mile from the village. The stone chapel of the sanctuary itself occupies a promontory, and is the second to serve in this place. An enormous parking lot and a primitive, cinder-block dormitory stand beside it (Figure 4.2).

The eighteenth-century statues of Cosma and Damiano usually reside in the *chiesa matrice* at the town center. On feast days, they are moved to the center of the church and then carried through the streets in several, solemn processions: a candlelight walk to mark the stations of the cross; a daytime journey to the local sanctuary; and on the following day, a procession back to the chiesa matrice. The statues reside overnight in the sanctuary.

Little Riace celebrates in a big way. Five thousand pilgrims will more than quadruple its population. In anticipation of their arrival, the main church was

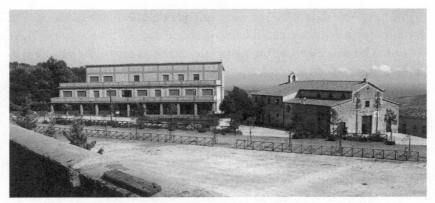

FIGURE 4.2 Hospice and sanctuary to santi medici, Riace, Calabria, Italy, 2001.

decked in elaborate cloth hangings with shiny gold and silver trim. Illuminations lined the streets. Midway amusements near the central piazza lured children to the merry-go-round and candy stalls. A booth inside the chiesa
matrice sold votive body parts in wax—hands, feet, heads, and breasts
(Figure 4.3). These items were like the anatomical objects found by archeologists in the Roman fountain of Juturna.

The sanctuary precinct appeared deserted, but we found Renzo Valilà
alone inside, seeing to final details. A surveyor in his thirties and father of two
young children, he was the current head of the local confraternity. Much of
the planning must be done by him and his friends in their spare time. "*È bene
e bruta!*" he said with a broad smile. When asked how old the tradition in
Riace is, he replied that it was at least a thousand years old and gave us a copy
of Pazzano and Capponi's scholarly history of the town. Documents in the
Vatican archives support his answer. Renzo found the switch to light the
sanctuary, which features three large, brightly colored canvases by the early
twentieth-century uncle-nephew team of Carmelo Zimatore and Diego
Grillo. In vivid realism, they show the saints healing, imprisoned, and dying.

Pilgrims come from far and wide, he told us; most will stay awake all night
as part of their sacrifice. Staying in a comfortable hotel nearby would not
count. He was not at all surprised that Hotel Federica had vacancies.

Many sick people attend the feast-day celebrations, praying for cures. The
cinder-block dormitory had to be constructed in haste just a few years earlier,
because of the growing number of infirm and elderly who could not tolerate
an entire night out-of-doors. Renzo knew that it was not pretty, but, he said,
funds were lacking for embellishments. It serves as adequate shelter on one or
two nights of the year. He took us back to the main church for an insider's

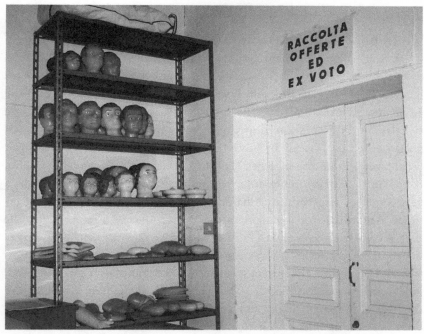

FIGURE 4.3 Wax votives for sale—heads, arms, breasts, eyes. Riace, Calabria, Italy, 2001.

tour and then offered us coffee. He would go to Torino soon. About twenty years ago, a group of people from Riace moved north for work and founded a feast-day celebration to the santi medici. His responsibilities included maintaining contact with them.

We asked about miracles. Yes, people claimed to obtain favors, he said. He seemed amused by the thought. As a skeptical scientist, his interest was in contributing to the tradition of his community; he served the confraternity because he felt that it was "his turn"—maybe he would continue for three years or so, probably no more. Someone else should take over. In this way, it would stay alive and ownership would be shared.

That night the chiesa matrice was packed. People spilled out the door and down the steps, craning to get a look at the glowing interior with its glittering backdrop for the saints. At the end of mass, the statues and relics were carried outside, a retinue of a hundred people assembled in the little piazza, lighting candles and chanting, and the procession slowly made its way through the town. The streets were lined with onlookers and the café had reopened. Every so often, the small parade would stop for prayers and to recall the stations of the cross. Some women fell on their knees, holding their rosaries in prayer.

San Cosmo Albanese (pop. 645)

We left Riace ahead of the wave of pilgrims and pressed on northeast up the Ionian coast of Calabria to San Cosmo Albanese, the hometown of the founders and celebrants of the Manhattan feast for the santi medici. The town occupies olive-grove hills, fifteen miles southwest of the archeological site of Sibaris. This ancient Greek city was founded in the eighth century BC and razed in 510 BC by its rival, nearby Croton. In this region especially, Greek and Byzantine influences still abound with unusual twists. From the fifteenth century following the Ottoman invasion, Albanian Christian immigrants renewed these traditions and brought a new language, Arbëresh, an Albanian dialect with Italian and Greek overtones. According to documents in the Vatican library, a sanctuary to the santi medici has been situated in these hills since at least 1089, but the existing church is modern.[12] The handsome, banana yellow exterior leaves visitors unprepared for the ornate spectacle of its Byzantine-inspired interior: golden mosaics and ceiling frescoes, painted in 1979, depict stories from the lives of the santi medici and the Bible (Figure 4.4). Was it the generosity of the emigrants to America that made this tiny town seem to exude

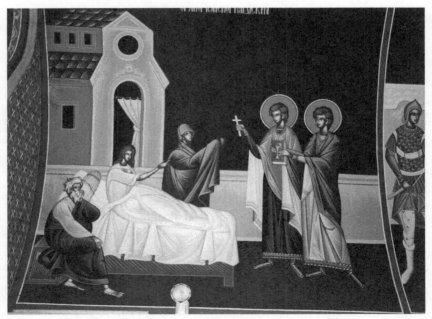

FIGURE 4.4 Ceiling painting of santi medici tending the sick, San Cosmo Albanese, Calabria, Italy.

wealth? A market had assembled around the church, but no pilgrims had yet appeared and the merchants were irritable and bored. To my surprise, this church and its festival seemed much more prosperous than its waning satellite in Manhattan, whose gifts it seemed to have absorbed with scant sign of acknowledgment.

Puglia

Every town in Italy has a church to the Virgin, or to Saint Peter, or Saint Francis, and it would be difficult, if not silly, to try to explain why. These holy people are famous and popular; of course, their veneration is widespread. Numerous though the santi medici shrines may be, most Italian towns do *not* have them. Only in Puglia may the reverse be true: there, almost every town has a church or chapel to Cosmas and Damian. Pierre Julien provided a list of more than forty place names (see Table 7). The extraordinary concentration of santi medici in Puglia demands some explanation. Plausible factors include the great antiquity and variety of its holy places: prehistoric, healing sanctuaries and troglodytic chapels hewn in the rock by the Ligurians and Celts, especially near Matera; extensive Greek settlements honoring the Dioscuri; lingering Byzantine influences; a member of the Medici family who favored the region; the arrival of relics; and the "contagious" veneration of favorite regional saints that spreads from one village to another. None of these potential factors can be proven or refuted.

The largest of these sites are in Bitonto and Alberobello. Pilgrims in Utica and Toronto knew of the Bitonto shrine. Settlers from Alberobello founded the Utica devotion, where the memory of homeland is still strong. A few Toronto pilgrims, originally from Barí, also recalled the Alberobello feast.

Alberobello (pop. 11,000)

Handsome forty-something Giovanni Sisto stands on the quai of the Alberobello train station, his station-master's red hat smartly in place. His colleague taps my shoulder and points between two nearby trees to a far-off hill. He holds up ten fingers, folding down one each second; as soon as the last finger is down, a train speeds across the distant hillside in the gap between the trees. The man grins, pleased to have impressed a foreigner with the punctuality of the Italian railway. Again he flashes up five fingers, and, indeed, precisely five minutes later, the train glides into the station. When it pulls out, the crowd disperses, and Giovanni is free to leave.

We came to Alberobello because it was the original home of the immigrant founders of Utica's veneration of the santi medici. But it is a UNESCO
world-heritage site for a completely different reason: its *trulli*, the white-
washed, beehive-shaped, stone dwellings. Their design is prehistoric, although
the oldest *trullo* still standing dates from the eighteenth century. Giovanni
lives in an expanded trullo with his university-educated wife, Lorita, who
teaches history and philosophy in the high school, and their two daughters,
Angela and Pieranna. Deacon Bill Dischiavo had given me the contact information for Giovanni, who was working in his spare time to complete his
degree in political science. The Sistos adopted us for our stay through the feast
of the santi medici, and they spoiled us with good food, good wine, good
company, and wild excursions. Everyone knows Giovanni.

Each year, thousands of tourists from all over the world come to Alberobello to see the trulli. Few visitors realize or care that the santi medici are the
town's patrons and that the weeklong celebration of their feast is a spectacular
example of the genre that Italians do so well. A 1930 article in the *National
Geographic* about the trulli included a photograph of the feast-day crowd
bearing statues of the unidentified saints.[13]

The tremendous influx for the *festa* derives mostly from the immediate
surroundings. Local historian and school teacher Angelo Martellotta traced
the Alberobello origins of veneration of Saints Cosmas and Damian to the
1630s, and a church that was dedicated to them in 1663.[14] He wrote how the
wife of a local count from Alberobello's feudal past had been particularly
devoted to the twins; however, the timing suggests that they may have had
something to do with the end of two great epidemics of plague that struck
Italy in the 1630s and the late 1650s. The polychrome, life-sized statues date
from the 1780s. Heavily bearded, these figures were the inspiration for their
counterparts in Utica. The confraternity that prepares the celebration was
founded in the nineteenth century. Relics—a piece of the arm of San
Cosma, a fragment of skull of San Damiano—were donated in 1803 by
Cardinale de Somalia. The basilica has been rebuilt and modified multiple
times, most recently in 1884, while embellishments continue into the present: odd murals of the saints' trial and passion painted in the chancel
during the 1920s; magnificent bronze doors representing the Beatitudes
erected in 1975; the stabilizing of the left tower in the 1980s; Papal designation as a Basilica Minore in 2000.

Preparations for the feast begin months in advance. The town is festooned
in colored lights on lattice arches over the streets, with different companies
competing for this honor and the citizens making comparisons from one year

to the next. Vendors set up booths for selling T-shirts, stockings, toys, dishes, knives, religious artifacts, and food along the main street. At these booths in 2001, Padre Pio was more in appearance than the santi medici; he would be canonized the following year. The lower town is invaded with midway rides and vendors of crafts and kitsch. The bandstand in the main square hosts a series of concerts every evening, and Verdi, Puccini, and Rossini enliven the cafes. We met Giovanni and family for ice cream and coffee in the piazza and they explained what would happen over the next few days so that we would miss none of the highlights.

On the morning of September 27, in keeping with Giovanni's instruction, I crawl out of bed at 3:30 a.m. In the cool dark, the streets are filled with padding footsteps and subdued voices moving steadily toward the piazza at the basilica steps. Giovanni and Lorita attend the early mass every year, and they are waiting at the prearranged corner. An altar has been set outside on the steps facing the main street, filled with a thousand or more pilgrims. Some are barefoot; they have walked ten or twelve miles through the night to arrive in time for this 4 a.m. mass, the first of hourly masses that will continue until 11 a.m. Some will stay to hear all seven masses before joining the daytime procession. It is an act of devotion. No one suggests that it is because of illness.

During the final mass late that morning, the priest makes a longer sermon and prays for the tragic losses of September 11 just two weeks earlier. He appeals for world peace and expresses sadness for absent friends, especially the Americans who normally come to Alberobello every year; their flights have been cancelled in the wake of the terrorist attacks. He prays for the sick too, but the tasks of the santi medici in Alberobello do not seem to be any more medical than those of other saints. I remember my idea that the twin saints have been hyper-medicalized in America.

Later that morning, Giovanni and I drop in on the headquarters of the confraternity organizing committee. The members are mellow and friendly; their feast is well launched and, so far, proceeding well. We ask about sick people, doctors, or others—they seem surprised. If there are healings, they are private. Once in a while, a doctor may join the confraternity, but of the 500 members of the *cavalieri* at present, they could think of only two who were health-care professionals: brothers—one a doctor, the other a pharmacist—like the saints! But they bear different surnames because of an error made at the registration of one birth. This tale seemed to be common knowledge, cherished for its quaint originality and its fraternal connection to the saints. The telling brought smiles and nods around the cramped office.

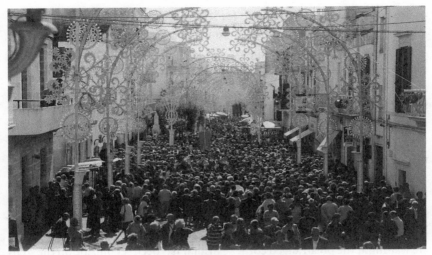

FIGURE 4.5 Daytime procession, Alberobello, Puglia, Italy, 2001.

After the late morning mass, the two statues are carried down the church steps and into the street (Figure 4.5). The priests and a visiting bishop lead the procession, bearing the relics and chanting prayers through a microphone. The statues are carried by the *cavalieri* of the confraternity wearing green and brown capes and organized in squads of six or eight. They take turns bearing first one statue for a hundred meters or so, and then the next statue. The distance between the two statues is lined on either side by cavalieri waiting for their next turn. A few cavalieri are women, an innovation that met some resistance a few years ago (Figure 4.6). At least two bands provide music, sometimes solemn, sometimes festive. The devout fall into a loose procession that takes more than two hours to complete its long circuit through many streets. Young and old alike participate. I notice more bare feet. Observers crowd the way, some walking beside the procession rather than in it. Others watch patiently from windows and balconies.

At midday, the Sisto family sits down to a massive meal, together with Lorita's sister, Margarita, her husband, Salvatore, and their three boys who have driven over from Locorotondo where they too live in a large, renovated trullo. Angela's friends are there too. The food keeps coming and coming. It is delicious. We learn that Lorita and Margarita are Albanese—and still speak that Arbëresh version of Italian, especially when they want privacy. They are amazed that we have been to San Cosmo Albanese, but the connection with their hometown's patron saints had never struck them before. Finding the conversation insufficiently entertaining, the young people turn

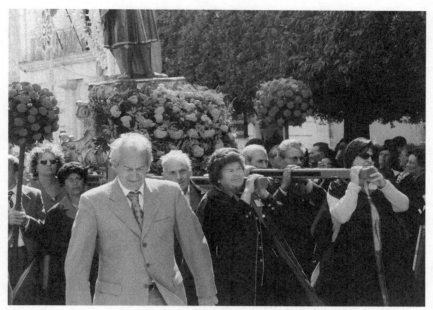

FIGURE 4.6 Women *cavalieri* carrying the statues, Alberobello, Puglia, Italy, 2001.

on the television to a loud music channel, and are chided to keep it down. They soon leave for the festivities in the streets. Pieranna and her cousins go to play with the kittens and the tortoise in the minuscule garden.

Giovanni and Lorita take me to meet the elderly Giorgio Citò and his son—photographers, collectors, archivists, and local historians par excellence. Their dimly lit atelier is a dusty, jumbled museum of books, paintings, and artifacts of every description. But Giorgio knows exactly where to find things in the apparent chaos. While his son works at a computer, Giorgio provides me with dozens of postcards that feature reproductions of historic photographs of the town. I recognize some of the images that had been printed in the 1930 *National Geographic*. He seems to know the date of every architectural and political change in the region. The veneration of the santi medici is deeply rooted here in Alberobello, but, again, the medical angle seems no more pronounced for them than for any other patron saints.

The talented Annese family has been photographing their town's feast for thirty years or more. Their business is owned and operated by four siblings—two brothers and two sisters, none married—specializing in weddings and portraiture. But the compelling color and drama of the feast appeals to their considerable artistry. Using Pierre Julien's name as an entrée results in a warm reception, archives opened and duplicate photographs generously given. They

show photographs of out-of-country visitors at an annual gathering that has
been cancelled this year because of the attacks in the United States. Months
later a fat envelope will arrive with choice reproductions of the events of 2001.

During the day, the basilica is open and many people wander in to pray, to
visit the tables where calendars, prayer cards, rosaries, and other objects of
devotion are free for the taking, although it is normal to leave an offering.
Most of these people are elderly women. Giovanni marches me into the vestry
at the back of the church and invades the private office of the tall distinguished priest, Don Giovanni Martellotta. Giovanni introduces himself,
although probably it is unnecessary, and me. He fires my questions at the
priest, who answers mechanically and looks tired from days of endless visitors; he hands us copies of church histories, as if to be rid of us. He pauses
when we ask if the doctor saints of Alberobello are medical, if their acts are
acts of healing. He looks worried, as if it might be a trick question. Not especially, he replies, no more than any other saint—and he cautions us that healing is a spiritual matter as much as it is physical. The festival caters to all
pilgrims, he said, not only to the sick.

In the early evening, another procession assembles. Once again the saints
are carried out of the basilica by the convoy of cavalieri, as the bishop and
priest take the lead with the relics, followed by the statues, and the bands. But
now the sinuous parade twinkles with lights of gigantic candles, three feet tall
and more than two inches thick. Some pilgrims carry the same candle year
after year. This procession takes a longer route that runs by the trulli in the
oldest part of town. Many more people participate: representatives from local
municipalities, other churches, and other confraternities. Salvatore represents
Locorotondo, because the mayor is unavailable, and he wears a *tricolore* sash.

After the statues pass, the bystanders tend to fall in behind and join the
procession. Darkness falls. Giovanni and I leave Margarita and Lorita in the
tail-end of the procession and dash through a side street into the town center
near the bandstand. We arrive in time to watch the priests pass through, followed by the officials; we catch Salvatore's bemused glance. Then as the first
statue arrives a loud explosion shatters the air, brilliant fireworks shimmer and
hiss—and a large, hot-air balloon, blazoned with an image of Cosmas, blasts
high into the atmosphere where it catches fire and shrivels in dust. Another
balloon is sent soaring when Damian's statue arrives. The dangerous launching
of these short-lived *montgolfiers* can be seen and heard all over town.

Much later, we gather on a friend's rooftop for the spectacular display of fireworks. The celebration is winding down. Lorita tells me she always feels a little
depressed when it is over. She likes the relaxed atmosphere, the combination of

religious and secular celebration, the visitors. The end of the feast signals the beginning of autumn and a slow school year. On this our last day, she wears an open neck blouse and I notice that, sometime in her life, Lorita's sternum was split—possibly an operation on her heart. Had the saints helped? I cannot ask, but I saw, and she knows (and probably intended) that I did. These gentle people remain our friends, sending news of their town every year. Giovanni completed his degree in 2005 and Angela is now an engineer.

Bitonto (pop. 56,000)

"La chiesa è aperta." We looked up. "La chiesa è aperta," the swarthy man repeated, pointing to the open door. We had been sitting in the sun in the wide piazza near the modern basilica of the Santi Medici at Bitonto (Figure 4.7). At our arrival, a visit was not possible because a wedding was going on inside the basilica. Wedding obstacles were becoming a major theme of the trip. Immediately after, it had closed for lunch. Thwarted again. In the sacristy, we had time only to glance at a spectacular collection of ex voto paintings and to purchase a previously unknown history book, before its shop closed too. We decided to wait through the long lunch break. I read the history on a bench outside; it was surprisingly well done.

For some time, the man had been pacing back and forth a few meters away, eyeing us with curiosity or suspicion. Slightly stout, with a stubble beard and an open collar, he looked harmless enough, but you can't be too careful with strangers. Somehow, this man sensed that we were waiting for the church to reopen. So, I left David on the bench and entered the basilica, slightly annoyed that the man followed more closely than was comfortable. His watching inhibited my contemplation of the interior—so I gave up and looked at him directly.

"Where are you from?" he asked. I told him.

"Why are you here?" I tried to explain.

"And you?"

He grinned and pointed to the book still in my hands. "I wrote that book."

Giuseppe "Pepe" Cannito is a historian, trained in Rome. So pleased and astonished was he to discover someone actually reading his work that he had to find out why. The santi medici of Toronto were new to him; it would be his pleasure to put them in a future edition and show me around the Bitonto sanctuary.

Bitonto claims to be the oldest and largest shrine devoted to Cosmas and Damian in all of Italy. It lies only thirty miles from Alberobello on the other

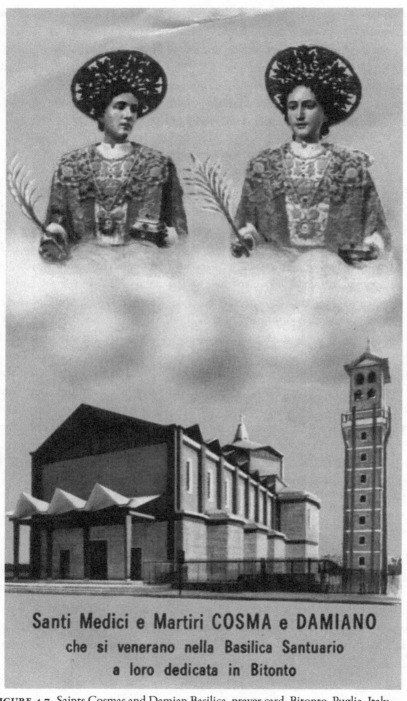

Santi Medici e Martiri COSMA e DAMIANO
che si venerano nella Basilica Santuario
a loro dedicata in Bitonto

FIGURE 4.7 Saints Cosmas and Damian Basilica, prayer card, Bitonto, Puglia, Italy.

side of Barí province, but the townsfolk of Bitonto seem to deny all knowledge of Alberobello (and vice versa). The feast-day celebrations in Bitonto
were moved from late September to the third week of October many years
ago so as not to interfere with the harvest. Avoiding conflicts with other local
festivals would surely have been another reason, but it is not acknowledged.
On feast days, as many as five thousand will gather in the square. That afternoon, a scant dozen people were praying in isolated spots throughout the basilica; bothered by our talking, several hissed at us to "shush."

The precise year of origin of the veneration in Bitonto is unknown, but
some objects hint at its age: a thirteenth-century mural (now in the local museum); a fourteenth-century bas relief of the twin saints (now in the altar of
the crypt); and two fifteenth-century statues, both from an older church that
was dedicated to Saint Luke, the physician. A chapel for the twin saints
appeared in the fifteenth century, but it was long in decline and abandoned
sometime after 1659. By 1676 the cult had been fully transferred to the church
of San Giorgio Martire, where the *festa* grew. New statues were acquired in
the eighteenth century. After several more enlargements, that church could
expand no further and yet it was not large enough for the popular devotion.

At the urging of Bishop Aurelio Marena, a large piazza on the edge of the
old town became the site of the new basilica, erected between 1958 and 1963,
known as the "Pompeii of Puglia."[15] A much older chapel had to be demolished to create the space, a "victim of topographical exigencies," wrote Pepe; if
this decision had been controversial, he did not record it.[16] Pope Paul VI recognized the new church as a Basilica Pontificia Minore in 1975. It has a free-
standing campanile and is decorated with many interesting pieces of art,
stained glass, mosaics, and a full-sized replica of Michelangelo's "Pietà."

Pepe demonstrated the differences of the eighteenth-century statues of
the saints above the altar in a glass case—one wearing red, the other green.
Damiano's eyes seem to follow the person standing below; Cosma looks elsewhere. Youthful and beardless, these statues are similar to the ones rejected by
the people of Utica who preferred bearded saints like those of nearby Alberobello. Was this an example of what Sigmund Freud had called "the narcis-
sism of small differences"? Subliminal but sustained rivalry between the two
Italian towns may have compounded the unacceptability of beardless statues
in America.

Under these Bitonto statues, at the center of the altar, are relics. Every day,
pilgrims come to touch them hoping for cures. The altar relics are said to be
arm bones—again! Legend holds that they were translated from Canosa in
the ninth century, after the sixth-century church to the *santi medici* was

destroyed. Cannito, however, disputes this tale. He suggests that they were a gift from Rome in the sixteenth century—a gift that may well have been prompted by Giulio de' Medici's becoming bishop of Bitonto in 1517. This reasoning is compelling, as the earliest document attesting to the existence of the relics dates from 1572.[17]

A remarkable collection of about a hundred vivid ex-voto paintings tells miracle stories in naïve, visual form. Most were images of healing—people in bed, on the operating table, bleeding in the street, often with doctors and always with the young, beardless, red and green saints hovering nearby. Some were signed and dated. The earliest seemed to be from around 1800. The most recent contribution was the work of a young girl who had had successful heart surgery in 1993. Since the late 1970s, historians have used documents such as these as precious sources on popular devotion, cultural practices, and social history.[18] They could be a valuable source for medical history too. Pepe reproduced a few in his book, mentioning without delving into their anthropological potential.[19] According to this unique, pilgrim-generated source, the Bitonto miracles were definitely medical. These pictures resembled visual representations of the very tales that I had heard in the surveys back home—whether they were real miracles or merely acts of grace.

Of all the sites in Italy, Bitonto connects the saints most directly to medicine, not only of the past but also of the immediate present. This connection seems to be strengthening in several different ways. Behind the basilica, Cannito showed me a small clinic, newly opened to receive young men with AIDS and cancer. Funds are provided through the state and privately. The facilities are bright and homey. Patients can sit on a breezy terrace in sight of palm trees and the sea. Several doctors offer services: some *gratis*; others charge regular fees. The two nurses on duty during my visit were young men on military service. With eleven patients, the clinic was full. Pepe pointed to the place where a much larger hospital will be built to extend this charitable work in physical healing.

Still following Pepe, I entered a modern office building. To my embarrassment, we barged into a boardroom where a meeting was in progress. Several men and women, some of them religious, were in the midst of planning the Tenth Annual Conference of Ethics in Medicine, held under the auspices of the medical saints at the University of Barí. The topic for October 6–7, 2001, was to be stem cell research; scientists and philosophers would attend from Milan, Rome, and Pavia. The organizers graciously forgave our intrusion and accepted Pepe's explanation for my presence. They asked me to write a few words of greeting in English for posting at their website and insisted that I sign with my title and address. As we left, one of the clerics grabbed my hand and kissed it. Begun in 1993, the Fondazione Opera Santi Medici Cosma e Damiano has established a prize called the Premio Nazionale "Santi Medici Cosma e Damiano." It reinvigorates devotion to the Anargyroi by recognizing substantial contributions to science. In 2001 the prize would go to stem-cell research as part of the conference. It continues: in 2010 the thirteenth prize went to three young women doctors working in the area of chronic pain, an "orphan disease" that needs more attention; the fourteenth prize will be announced in the spring of 2013.[20]

In Bitonto, as in Howard Beach, New York, the saints' medical characteristics are emphasized. The many ex-votos, the clinic, the planned hospital, and the scientific conferences all tilted at physical healing and they endorsed human efforts to promote it. My theory of a more medical aspect to the North American devotion was exploded.

Campania—The Gulf of Salerno

"*Posso?*" Natale Persico asked, pulling out a chair. Not waiting for a reply, he sat down and leaned across the table, grinning, his white hair pulled tightly back in a skinny ponytail, his big hands folded, and his piercing eyes devouring us with intent curiosity. We had just staggered out of the Val de Ferriere to the village of Pogerola, smoldering in the unnatural October heat. From this improbable perch, dizzyingly high above the Amalfi Coast, sea and sky merged into a homogenous hot blue haze. Natale served us cool water and *limone* with the vigor of an Italian Zorba before launching into his interrogation. He seemed blithely unoffended by our poor grasp of his language. Where were we from? Why did we come? How far had we walked? His *taverna* was empty; the awnings and tablecloths stirred in the hot air. The solitude permitted broken replies and invited more questions.

This dashing, worldly man had been born in the house across the road. He had never lived anywhere else, was not married now or ever; he insisted we take his picture and with it, find him "una bella donna canadese." His modest business had perked up when an English travel writer mentioned it favorably. Incredulous that we had never heard of that book and managed to find him anyway, he promptly deflated, as if we had just trounced him in a round of his favorite game. As a lad, he went to school in Amalfi. He used to walk the 325 meters straight down and back up every day. Pogerola children now had a primary school, but for high school, they too must descend to Amalfi in the comfort of a bus. If they want university or medicine, they must go to Naples.

Not Salerno, I asked? He replied that some do go to Salerno, but that medicine at Naples is better because it is bigger and "much, much older."

Natale's information struck a discordant note. Salerno is the site of the
earliest medical "school" in all Europe, originating sometime in the ninth or
tenth century. Situated thirty-five miles south of Naples, in the embrace of a
vast, sunny gulf open to south and west, Salerno was at first Etruscan, before
becoming a Roman trading center at a crossroads of cultures. The Greek city
of Paestum, on the coastal plain further south, had flourished from 600 BC
until the decline of the Roman Empire. Among its many temples was an
Asklepion, dedicated to the Greek god of medicine. To the north, Pompeii,
an equally old city, predated Greek settlement and then basked in the glory of
Rome until that fateful explosion in AD 79. Its baths were large and well
known, and it too boasted a temple to Asklepios.

In the early ninth century, Salerno became the provincial capital under
Lombard domination. Immigration led to a blending of two cultures: from
nearby Amalfi to the west and Eboli to the southeast, and from distant Lom-
bardy in the north.[21] As befit a prominent city, medieval Salerno had an *ospedale*
and several learned physicians, whose existence is known from records describing their consultations for the affluent sick. One of the earliest, from 870,
concerns a doctor Gerolamo, who was consulted by a desperate young husband
from Rheginna Maiori, near Amalfi, for grave illness in his bride; Gerolamo is
said to have searched for a cure in "immensa volumina librorum."[22]

Together with much of southern Italy and Sicily, Salerno came under Norman rule with the 1076 conquest by Robert Guiscard, cousin of William who
had conquered England at Hastings ten years earlier. Contact with Sicilian
centers such as Monreale explains the pronounced Islamic aspects of the art
and architecture. Reflecting these multiple influences, legend has it that the
medical school at Salerno had four mythic founders: a Greek, a Roman, a Jew,
and a Saracen.[23] After two centuries of teaching, it was officially institutional-
ized in 1231, and its statutes published in 1280. By the fourteenth century, it
was already said to be losing status to its rival in Naples (founded in 1224),
although some scholars point to a sixteenth-century revival. The master narrative implies that Salerno's medical decline was due to its preferential shift
toward arcane, theoretical commentary and away from its original focus on
the pragmatics of clinical practice. But the school was not actually closed
until four centuries later, in 1811, when Napoleon set out to reorganize public
education. A new university opened in 1970; it now boasts a medical school.
Nothing remains of its medieval buildings, but libraries across Europe hold
manuscripts containing the school's wisdom, some in multiple copies.

Salernitan doctors, including a few women, wrote on uroscopy, surgery, gynecology, and health. The most famous of these documents is the much reproduced, much expanded, and much commented upon poem, the *Regimen sanitatis salernitanum*. They also interpreted ancient medical authors, Hippocrates and Galen. The eleventh-century Monte Cassino monk and Tunisian physician Constantine the African began translating Greek and Arab medical texts into Latin, expanding the sources available to Salerno doctors and those at other centers. His work was incorporated in the *Articella*, or standard teachings of the school.

The question has been asked many times why Salerno should have Europe's first medical school. Answers point to the ferment of influences, political, cultural, religious, and intellectual. But a medical school arises out of a concentration of doctors, and doctors gravitate to the sick. The presence of independent doctors and valuable libraries as early as the ninth century suggests that they may have followed prospective patients or the wealthy patrons who had been attracted to the region for its healthful properties. For example, spas apparently favored by the Roman elite included hot springs at Vesuvius and along the mountainous Amalfi Coast, which extends out from Salerno as the north-west arm of the gulf.

The relationship between religion and medicine of the Salerno school has been examined several times. The early medical professors were priests or monks and the relative proximity of Monte Cassino abbey (sixty miles north of Naples, ninety miles from Salerno) ensured a dialogue between scholars in church and those in academe. The writings and translations of Constantine the African pervaded medicine, but medicine seems to have had a reciprocal influence on religion here and elsewhere. For example, the crypt of the cathedral at Anagni, between Naples and Rome, is decorated with astonishing thirteenth-century frescoes, including Hippocrates, Galen, a cosmology, and a rendition of the four elements. To evoke the equivalent, imagine a mural in a church of our own time featuring two Nobel laureates, a stylized view of the human genome, and the periodic table of the elements. Medicine and religion were close, and some physicians and clerics—especially those in the vicinity of Salerno—celebrated that compatibility.

How could I not have Salerno in mind when visiting the Cosmas and Damian sanctuaries of Campania? From the center of the exquisite town of Ravello (pop. 2,500), high on a broad plateau opposite Natale's village of Pogerola, a footpath twists and turns down hundreds of steps to a narrow road, which winds like a shelf, partway down the cliff face. Past a bar and a fountain, another short flight leads up to a massive, rocky overhang that shelters the

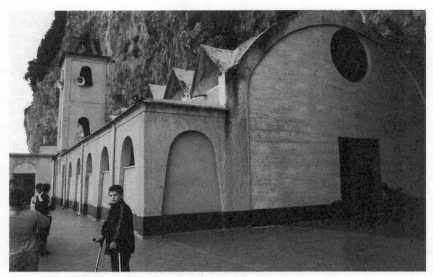

FIGURE 4.8 Sanctuary to the medical saints, Ravello, Campania, Italy, 2001.

sanctuary of the santi medici. Ravello is a famous tourist destination, but this sanctuary, halfway down the cliff, seems to cater only to locals (Figure 4.8).

A busload of visitors from nearby Maiori (pop. 5,600)—formerly Rheginna Maiori—were still in the church, having heard mass. Some were kneeling in silent meditation, others lit candles before the golden, reliquary busts, or they bought prayer cards and newsletters. A young boy on crutches mingled with the stragglers who were looking at several collections of ex-votos of cut metal and photographs that had been framed for display. The back walls were decorated with glittering mosaics installed in the 1990s, which were gigantic reproductions of the predella paintings of Cosmas and Damian by Fra Angelico in Florence's Convento San Marco: the miracle of the black leg, the trial and execution.

The sun was setting in a pink haze. From the balcony terrace, the wide sweep of the gulf lay below and beyond the next headland of Capo d'Orso; lights began to twinkle at Salerno some seven miles east for a crow or a boat—much further for a car. The attendant was closing up for the night but paused to chat.

The chapel had to be rebuilt in the 1960s, he said, because of heavy damage in the war. Without knowing the date of its founding, however, he insisted—of course—that it was the "first" and "oldest" Cosmas and Damian sanctuary in all Italy. Many healing miracles were worked here, and the group from Maiori had been praying for cures. Busloads of pilgrims came every day. He seemed amazed that I did not know. Had that young man, also from Maiori more than a millennium ago, brought his bride to this shrine before consulting the learned doctor in Salerno?

We passed motor scooters parked at the Santi Medici Bar as we climbed back up to Ravello's town center. Towering pine trees in the silky, evening light made the gleaming stone parvis an outdoor extension of its Duomo. The bronze doors were open. We went in to admire the fabulous mosaic pulpit and other stone work. Founded in 1086, the church is dedicated to Saint Pantaleon. A third-century martyr, like the santi medici, Pantaleon of Nicodemia had been a doctor too. In a chapel on the left of the main altar is a miraculous reliquary vial filled with his blood. Behind the chapel, a small space provides a closer view of the relic through a grill. The liquefaction of this blood relic is another wonder peculiar to the region, like that of San Gennaro and other saints in the Naples area.[24]

I began to find medical saints everywhere along the Amalfi Coast. Was it because of the Salerno school? Did it bespeak an ancient health industry in the region that long antedated the university? Was it merely wishful thinking? Would I have noticed as many medical saints had I looked anywhere else? Saint Luke the Evangelist, another physician, was the patron of Praiano a bit further west. The existing church was from 1588 and restored in the eighteenth century, but it claims to occupy an earlier structure going back to 1123, also dedicated to the physician apostle. The town celebrates his feast on October 18. Saint Vitus had been the patron of a local monastery at Positano; he too was a third-century martyr, who died in southern Italy and is said to have effected miraculous cures. The patron of epileptics, his name is associated with the movement disorder chorea, also known as Saint Vitus' Dance. The attribution derived from early modern forms of his veneration in northern Europe that entailed dancing before his image.[25]

The cathedral of Amalfi (pop. 5,500), dating from 959–1004, had originally been dedicated to the santi medici. When returning crusaders brought the relics of Saint Andrew, disciple of Christ and patron of Scotland, the building was expanded to the south and the designation of protector was changed to advertise the famous new relics. But a large chapel to the right of the chancel is lined with dozens of reliquary busts, arranged in three tiers. Those of Cosmas and Damian are front and center, on either side of the altar; they are said to date from the original church.

Could the sanctuary of Ravello, halfway up the cliff, have been a satellite or relic of the original Amalfi patrons—simply a dramatic place to honor local saints? Or by repeatedly choosing doctor saints were the clerics in the ninth and tenth centuries consciously catering to regional pride in medicine or the enterprise of serving sick travelers who needed spiritual care as well as physical?

These thoughts stuck with me for years. It seemed that both the Salerno medical school and the large number of doctor saints in that region might have been prompted by a preexisting market: the heavy concentration of wealthy, health pilgrims who had been flocking to that coast for its atmosphere and abundant food since antiquity and long before the advent of Christianity. A phrase oft used in teaching diagnostics is attributed to bank robber Willy Sutton: "Go where the money is." Obeying Sutton's Law, both the physicians and the saints had simply followed the sick. These musings about supply and demand involving saints and physicians eventually became the sixth paper from the project.[26]

Eboli (pop. 36,100)

On the other side of Salerno, a short distance south and east, lies Eboli, home to yet another shrine to the santi medici. Carlo Levi's book *Christ Stopped at Eboli* borrowed the title from a saying of the inland peoples of the southern *mezzogiorno*, who saw their mean surroundings as a sign of God's disinterest. The day that we arrived, Eboli indeed looked like Providence had relinquished his progress somewhere short of its gates. The *centro storico* was virtually abandoned, disconnected from the bustling, unattractive modern town below. Its castle is now a soft penitentiary where some inmates, at least, have the freedom to come and go. In 1980 a massive earthquake destroyed large parts of the town, killing 2,700. A building boom is underway and has created a fine museum that was still devoid of visitors, while trucks and cranes were hard at work turning the crumbling structures into livable spaces.

Just behind the *castello* prison is a huge, modern sanctuary dedicated to Cosmas and Damian. Enormous stained-glass windows, made in Florence, portray their miracles and passion in angular expressionist style. Flat, marble floors gleam in their reflected light. Subdued art-deco-style mosaics of the saints with sick people in wheelchairs line the walls. An older and much smaller church stands nearby.

The popular veneration of the santi medici at Eboli is said to have begun at around the year 1000 with Greek immigrants. The original church was destroyed in the late twelfth century, then rebuilt as the still-standing smaller church under the protection of Saint Sebastian. But the cult to the santi medici was revived in the late eighteenth century and its growing popularity led to the new sanctuary, which opened in 1957. On feast days, large crowds gather, some arriving to spend the night; wire fences and signs with directions to toilets hint at their numbers. But that afternoon, the doors opened nearly an hour late and occasional visitors were unhappy-looking men who paused just inside the door for a quiet moment and then left. Were they prisoners? And did the Eboli version of the saints extend to care for the incarcerated?

Isernia (pop. 21,100)

Ersilia Jannetta of Toronto, feast-day founder and donor of the santi medici statues in that city, hails from the spectacularly mountainous region of Campobasso province in the interior lands of Molise. As a girl, she had attended the celebrations of Cosmas and Damian in Isernia just to the west. That memory, as much as the compelling example of Utica, had prompted the donation to her Canadian parish. According to historian Angelo Martellotta, Isernia's devotion to the medical saints originated in 1130.[27]

It was late morning when we arrived and parking was impossible. Midday diners were filling the restaurant terraces while a splendid wedding was taking place in the cathedral. Golden, reliquary busts of the santi medici stood off to the right of the chancel, a velvet pouch for donations hanging from each (Figure 4.9). They smiled indulgently on the bride and groom, while the

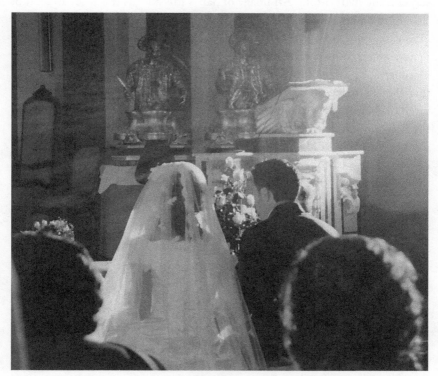

FIGURE 4.9 Wedding in cathedral with reliquary busts for the santi medici, Isernia, Molise, 2001.

organist-singer, an impressive young mezzo, offered one exquisite Handel aria after another. I did not have the nerve to approach the chancel. Men in their finery loitered on the porch outside, smoking, joking, and giving themselves collective permission to skip the ceremony and its music.

I asked people outside how the feast-day celebrations "worked" in Isernia. After a couple of false starts, interrupted by consultations and good-natured argument, they agreed on a reply. The golden busts are carried in a candlelit procession to the sanctuary, where they stay overnight; then they are brought back. Yes, sick people sometimes attend. Where was the sanctuary? An elegant, young man walked me to a railing and pointed to a building about a half mile away in the valley below.

Set behind the local hospital, on a little knoll covered in tall pines, the Isernia sanctuary to the santi medici was silent and empty, but drenched in warm incense as though a person-less service had ended moments before. Nearby lay a vast parking lot and a monastery with the tawdry air of a barrack. The sanctuary is old and lavishly decorated with pale frescoes in poor condition, depicting the lives and miracles of the saints—the black leg, the bosom serpent, the martyrdom. An image of San Vitus adorns the apse; an icon of the virgin hangs above the altar. Small statues of the santi medici repose in a glass case. How does this chapel relate to site of the modern hospital a few meters away? Which came first, the chapel or the hospital? A letter sent in October 2001 asking for more information received no reply. Some contend that the sanctuary sits on the site of an ancient pagan temple possibly dedicated to Priapus, the god of virility. This disputed "discovery" is attributed to the Scottish antiquarian and diplomat William Hamilton (1731-1803), who went to Isernia but did not attend the feast, after he was shown votive objects of erect penises. Modern guidebooks rely on a nineteenth-century description of the Isernia celebration as a by-now-familiar continuity of pagan rites with Saint Cosmas as "the modern Priapus." [28]

Santena (pop. 10,200)

Immigration had been a significant force in the North American sites, but it emerged as a factor within Italy too. Renzo Valilà had given us the phone number of his friend Damiano Gruttaroti in Santena, near Turin. By 1953 people from Riace had moved north for work in the factories, taking the santi medici with them. In 1965 they established the *Associazione dei santi martiri Cosma e Damiano* with the explicit goal of keeping alive the tradition of their hometown.[29] Damiano was currently serving as president. In April, toward the end of our sabbatical leave, Anita Johnston joined us for a week, and, of course, she was obliged to chase the saints too. We visited Santena and headed straight for the cathedral. But a thorough inspection of the premises revealed no chapels, no statues, and no mention of the twins—of course, the feast *was* five months away. Speaking Italian on the phone is not my favorite thing, but David dialed the number and handed me his phone. Damiano answered the phone in a friendly manner, then fetched his daughter, Beatrice, who spoke French. Once they understood that we were already in the piazza in front of the cathedral, they said "*Aspetti, aspetti!*" I was worried that they would not be able to recognize us, but ever pragmatic, Anita said that we were obvious. A short time later, a beautiful young woman approached us, saying, "*Salve.*" Beatrice wore black because her mother had died not long before. In-person communication, with hand gestures and facial expressions, is so much easier than the telephone.

She led us away from the cathedral and off the piazza into a school court-yard. At the end of the courtyard was a modest locked door under a hand-let-tered sign with palm branches, a crown, and an axe, bearing the words "SS Cosmae et Damiano martiribus dicatum A.D. MCMLXV." This modest room was the transplanted shrine of Riace migrants. Why was it not in the cathedral? Beatrice shrugged and explained that this displacement was an Italian class issue at work. Immigrant workers from the south were not entitled to decide what happened in the splendid cathedrals of the north. Here the Riace immigrants centered their devotion to the santi medici, and from here they marked the feast each year in a way that repeated the gestures of home: procession, statues, mass. The celebration involves the church as the statues are decorated, taken from the sanctuary, and carried through the streets accompanied by the priests, after which a mass is said in the main church.

Films of the feast-day events at Santena, Sferrocavallo, Riace, and else-where can now be found on *youtube.com*, making it possible to involve the folks back home or far away. Would I have done all this traveling if that had been possible in 2001? Would I have learned as much?

Rome, and the First Book

A few years earlier, Giulio Silano had charged that the miracles of my feast-day pilgrims, described in Chapter 3, were not really miracles in the strict sense of the word. One "official" miracle was already familiar from my hema-tology work in the cause of Marie Marguerite d'Youville: it was strongly med-ical, and it had been squared with the best science of our time.

But what were all the other miracles? The Vatican might have records about miracles in other places—in letters, diplomatic reports, special investigations—but the canonization process promised a reliable supply of so-called real miracles—if one could find and examine the files. Other historians had already pointed to the potential of the untapped source of cultural history in the thousands of depositions, like the *Positio super miraculo*, given me by Père Bouchaud.[30] A few scholars had applied several of these documents and other miracle stories to their work on specific times, places, or saints.[31] But no one seemed to have attempted an overview through time, and that is what I wanted to know. To answer Silano's concern, I wondered if it would be possible to continue chasing miracles, as the recognized deeds of saints, in the canonization records of the Vatican Secret Archives.

I planned a one-week visit in December 2001 as an academic tourist, simply to see if I would be allowed to consult the records and how far I could get. David went back to Geneva, and I took a room in a cheap hotel near the Termini train station.

After showing my passport and a letter from my dean, I was amazed to be granted permission to use the Archives with very few questions asked. Once the archivist understood my quest, he explained how to target the relevant files. I had made a list of all the saints canonized up to the year 2000 from 1588, when the rules were revised in the Counter Reformation; however, I intended to focus on the most recent causes, fearing that I would not understand the earlier records in terms of handwriting or medicine. The Archives, however, are sealed for the six most recent papacies—this meant 1922 when I first visited and later moved to 1939 following the death of John Paul II.

The indexes, or finding aids, were meticulous. Organized alphabetically by saints' names and subdivided by the type of document, they listed files for biography, virtues, miracles, and so on. Once I had found the call number for a miracle file, I could fill out a paper slip as a requisition, and the corresponding *busta* would appear, usually within thirty minutes. But consultation was limited to only three files a day, and the third file could not be requested until after the first had been returned.

Already on the first day, I examined miracle files from three different saints: Angela Merici (canonized in 1807), Joan of Arc, and Gabriel of the Sorrowful Virgin (both canonized in 1920). Angela had interceded in 1781 for twenty-nine-year-old Maria d'Aquafreddo, who suffered what seemed like a stroke with convulsions, loss of speech and right-sided paralysis, although it could have been hysteria in our time. Appeals to Joan of Arc preceded the healings of tuberculous peritonitis in a seventeen-year-old girl at Lyons in

1909 and of an infected, ulcerated heel in a married woman from Orleans in 1910; witnesses in both cases were interrogated in 1911. Gabriel was credited with repairing the inguinal hernia of a twenty-nine-year-old man from Gallipoli in 1912. Just like my *positio* on the Ottawa leukemia cure, these files contained the verbatim testimony of all the witnesses to each miracle, doctors too—with their names, ages, training, and income.

The Vatican Secret Archives closes every day at 1 p.m., although it is open six days a week. The archivists explained how I could also use the Vatican Library, next door, in the afternoons. Book orders in the library had to be placed before noon, but I could leave the archive briefly once each morning, place my book orders there, and return to finish off my three archival files. By the time the archive closed, the maximum of five books would be waiting at the library for an afternoon's study until 5:30 p.m., when it closed too. Both archival files and books could be set aside for another day if I did not manage to finish in one sitting. Many of the more recent *positiones* had been printed and bound as books, just like the one that Père Bouchaud had given me back in 1990. As a result, miracles could be found in the library too, and these primary-source documents were not bound by date restrictions. It was therefore possible, through the library, to learn of miracles more recent than the cutoff dates of 1922 or 1939.

The work slipped into a steady rhythm fed by obsession and joy. I'd take bus number 64 from the Termini to arrive at the archive for its opening. Then I'd work all morning, skip lunch, and work all afternoon in the library. At night, I would buy a panini and some fruit at the vendors near the train station and transcribe my penciled scrawl into a database to keep track of all the different bits of information. That monastic process served to embed the stories in my mind, and it suggested other questions and strategies.

At the end of the first week, I had details on forty-four miracles pertaining to twenty-one saints, canonized from 1807 to 1991. Only two miracles were not healings. Both were attributed to Clara of the Cross of Montefalco: one was her incorrupt corpse—she had died in 1308; the other was an expulsion of demons, which had happened long before 1726 when the testimony was gathered. Clara's corpse had been studied on several occasions since her death, and it has been the object of scholars since her canonization.[32] The same file also contained many other miracles of a healing nature, nine of which I transcribed into the database with the rest.

Medicine was intimately connected to these stories in this first collection. The people of the forty-two healing miracles had all been seen by doctors before they appealed to the candidates for sainthood. But even the *miraculé* possessed by demons and the corpse of Santa Clara had also been examined by physicians. Each evening I went back to my hotel on Bus 64, exhausted but ecstatic that I had been let into that famous, sacred place, and relieved that the files were so easy to use. These cases did not seem to be qualitatively different from the kinds of stories told to me by pilgrims at the feast days.

I went back to Rome for a second week's research in May 2002, choosing the same cheap hotel and adding to my database another fifty-eight miracles worked by thirty-six more saints, canonized or beatified from 1747 to 1977. Some files contained two or more miracles, making it possible to gather many more than three in a single day. Again, all but two miracles in this week's work were healings from physical illness; most contained medical testimony of treating doctors and expert witnesses. I began to realize that these depositions not only chart miracles of different eras, but bear witness to the perceived limits of scientific knowledge.

This part of my amorphous project took on a life of its own. Over the next seven years, I would make eight increasingly long trips to Rome to gather as many miracles as possible. I expanded my criteria from the most recent canonizations to include at least one miracle from every canonization since 1588. No longer preoccupied by answering Silano's criticism, I was interested in the files as a source of medical history: how the diagnoses changed through time, what treatments were used, how the doctors reacted, and how up-to-date was their science.

The cheap hotel near Termini gave way to small apartments in the much nicer *centro storico*, rented on the Internet and paid for upon jet-lagged arrival with a fistful of euros. Every new dwelling had its charms and its flaws, but the privacy offered blessed release from the bus and the chain-smoking, bleary-eyed hotelier back at Termini. They fed the attractive illusion of making a life in the eternal city. Every night, I ate in and toiled on the database over glasses of red wine.

Cosmas and Damian were not to be found in these canonization files. Because they were early martyrs, they had never been subjected to the process that developed with the foundation of the Congregation of Rites in 1588. Nevertheless, the odd miraculé in my collection had appealed to the santi medici first, before turning to the new, would-be saint; in those cases, the holy twins may have failed, but it was significant that they had been consulted in time of medical need.

Many saints are associated with various diseases and infirmities because they suffered similar ailments or brutal torture—like saints Lucy (eyes) and Agatha (breasts)—at the time of their death.[33] But at least sixty-five physicians, hospital founders, or healers are recognized as saints, born from the first century to the twentieth (Table 8).[34] Some are venerated by medical associations with online calendars.[35]

Of the eighteen post-Congregation saints or blesseds who were once doctors or hospital founders, most were recognized recently: seven in the nineteenth century, seven in the twentieth- or twenty-first centuries. Only two, Moscati and Molla, were laypeople; the others were in religious orders. I read eighteen of the miracles attributed to them: all were healings of physical disease; however, two of those attributed to the thirteenth-century Filippo Benizi were resurrections, "cures" of death.

I also looked in the archives and libraries for more information about the history of the geographic sites of devotion to the santi medici that I had visited earlier in the year to determine when or why the designations were established. But few documents prior to the year 1000 have survived, and those that are accessible and indexed pertain to large cities and important people. For the history of hamlets and villages, we must choose to believe the local historians—or not. But which ones? Only a single site can be the oldest.[36] Nevertheless, it was instructive to recognize that the numerous priority claims to being the first or the oldest site were also claims to authenticity and pride.

While in Rome, I often visited the basilica to the santi medici. One Saturday in December 2001, a wedding was taking place despite a cluster of tourists; the white limo stood on the porch giving on to the Via dei Fori Imperiali. While waiting, I gazed out past the ancient rotunda behind the nave to the forum, with the ruins of the temple to Castor and Pollux, and the fountain of Juturna, where cures were worked and votives left. On another day, a woman in a wheelchair was being helped to light candles at the edge of the chancel under the great mosaic. This narrow precinct of the eternal city has been dedicated to medicine and religion for more than 2,500 years.

At one time, Saints Cosmas and Damian had been patrons of eight churches in Rome. But all that remain now are the great basilica and the San Cosimato church in Travestere with its much damaged monastery. I went to San Cosimato too. The porch, church, and two cloisters with their ruddy walls and unruly garden can still be visited. Despite their state of poor repair, they enclose a modern medical service specialized in geriatrics. Exciting as it was to find health-care provision in a former Cosmas and Damian convent, it is important not to read too much into the succession of their monastery by a hospital; most monasteries and convents of Europe also catered to the sick, regardless of who had been invoked as their patron saints.[37]

It would be wrong to suggest that these studious sojourns were devoid of fun and companionship; I met some wonderful people. Anne Overell from Leeds asked me in cultivated Italian, "*Scusi, dov'è il bagno?*" and I enjoyed being able to offer directions to "the Ladies" of the Vatican Archives. During her stay, we did coffee most days with the ghostly company of her good heretics. Elizabeth A. (Peggy) Brown, the feisty president of the Society for Medieval Studies, was hot on the trail of a French queen; she was more grateful for a few scraps of information from my database than the service merited, but I took heart from her verve. A handsome Franciscan sat beside me in the library one afternoon, poring over a photograph. I loved his rough habit, the thick rope about his waist, his dark eyes, and bare, sandaled feet—in winter. Did I imagine that he kept glancing my way? Finally, our eyes locked, and he leaned over to ask, "*Lei è paleografista?*" inviting me to examine the utterly indecipherable inscription lying on the table. "*No,*" I managed. "*Mi dispiace; sono canadese.*" He shrugged, smiled, and turned back to his photograph, fully accepting a world divided into paleographers and Canadians. I have seen him often since that first encounter; we are both graying, and he can't quite place me, but always remembers that I am from Canada.

Then there was the bus strike. It didn't affect me, as I could walk to the Vatican each day. But Steve Andes, an American grad student at Oxford, was apoplectic that his precious week would be ruined if the busses stopped, because he had taken cheap-as-possible accommodations far from the Vatican. To keep up his work on the Jesuits in Latin America, Steve spent two nights on the miserable, folding sofa in my little apartment. I don't think he slept much because he was allergic to something, maybe the mold in the stone walls. Petite Madre Sonia Sapena also became my friend one day as we both waited to renew our archival passes. In the cause for canonization of her founder, she had been sent from Valencia to Rome seeking information about her religious order to compensate for the missing records burned in the civil war. An inveterate e-mailer and a whiz with digital photography, she is now in a secluded retreat back in Spain.

The *signori* in the Archives were invariably courteous and never was a file missing. Once I managed to make a joke in halting Italian by suggesting that the trick of how to work the temperamental pencil sharpener was the *real* secret of the Secret Archives. It so pleased one of the *signori* that he told the others and they spent the morning smiling approvingly. At noon on the last open day before Christmas 2003, they brought me a requisition for an exceptional fourth file as a *regalo di Natale* and they let me take their picture. I was sorry when the work was done.

By 2008 I had information on 1,400 miracles, and Oxford University Press published my book the following year. The whole thing was a long tangent from the original quest to explain the santi medici.

COSMAS AND DAMIAN were celebrated throughout Europe from a very early date. The churches in Rome and Constantinople were well known and gifts (or thefts) of relics served to spread and deepen the devotion in other places. Crusades, colonization, and convent care of the sick extended their cult.

In terms of theory, the trip to Europe confirmed the role of diffusion in the founding of several sites of veneration beyond, and even within, Italy—Isernia for Toronto, Gaeta for Cambridge, Alberobello for Utica, Riace for Santena. Nostalgia for homeland and national identity were related to that diffusion. A possible rivalry between Alberobello and Bitonto exemplifies the local nature of identity, and recapitulates the imitative aspects of the devotions in Toronto and Utica.

The sociological view that the saints and their feast days filled important social functions was also supported by observations in the many sites we visited. The exact nature of these roles varied from place to place—and may also have changed through time within each place. Along these lines, the patterns of veneration in the New World stray from the originals. For example, the Italian feasts of Alberobello, San Cosmo de Albanese, and Riace were much larger than their offspring, while that of the descendant in Cambridge, Massachusetts, overshadows its progenitor in Gaeta. The explicit emphasis on medicine, science, and research, found at Howard Beach, was not unique to North America, especially given the activities in Bitonto. The purpose of the events clearly shifted through time and probably altered back in the Old World too after the departure of emigrants.

But the other theories could not be refuted, nor did they find much support. For example, the genealogical view that the medical twins of the Catholic Church might be connected to the ancient Dioscuri must remain unproven. True, geographic overlap of their cults in some places is undeniable, but the absence of any records for at least a millennium leaves unrefuted the contradictory possibilities of both continuity and hiatus. Somehow, religious opposition to that notion is fading. Significantly, one of the guidebooks to the Roman basilica refers directly to the Castor and Pollux temple as a reason for the deliberate choice of location in the sixth century.[38]

Intriguing though it was that so many sites claimed to be the "oldest" in Europe or in Italy, none could establish the claim with certainty. Records identifying dates of origin tilt toward specific moments of saintly revival through triggers, such as gifts of relics, recovery from epidemics, the presence of medical schools, and the founding of professional societies. Each of these events could simply have injected new life in preexisting, local devotion. Or, to the contrary, they could have marked the sudden abandonment of old traditions in favor of a new devotion.

As for the sophisticated, psychoanalytical view, again consolation and comfort seem plausible, but could be neither confirmed nor denied. My surveys of pilgrims might be said to have produced some evidence in that direction, if they could be counted on for accuracy—and we had some worries about that. Support for this psychoanalytic theory would eventually come from an unimagined source back home in North America.

After all that time in the Vatican archives and library, I could now at least reply with confidence to Giulio Silano: the "miracles" described by the feast-day pilgrims were qualitatively similar to the "real" miracles of the theologians. They were events that could not be explained by science, at least in the moment of their investigation; however, there could be no doubt that they had occurred, whether they had been caused by God or something else. And all these miracles—official and unofficial—were medical. Wherever and whenever they were consulted, Cosmas and Damian, and possibly all the other saints too, were deeply engaged in health care. Did my medical colleagues know?

Miracles, Medicine, and MEDLINE

Prayer indeed is good, but while calling on the gods a man
should himself lend a hand.
—HIPPOCRATES, *Regimen IV, LXXXVI. Trans. W. H. S. Jones, Hippocrates, 4: 423.*

DURING OUR TIME in Europe, Julia Cataudella had continued the surveys, although she was well launched in her family medicine residency. But for all her cultural closeness to these pilgrims in their Italian language and shared religious faith, she, too, found it awkward to do the work. Placing survey sheets at the back of the Toronto church did not result in many responses, possibly owing, the priest suggested, to relative illiteracy among parishioners. She wrote about this discomfort in her diary in September 2002: "I had a bit of trouble doing the survey; felt somehow it wasn't appropriate," especially in the context of the "sense of reverence in the pilgrims." She noted that it was easier to talk to people who remained outside the church—rather than those who had been inside. Astutely, she wondered if this preference would inadvertently skew results away from the most devoted.

Father Stefano, one of the Toronto priests, welcomed Julia and helped find willing subjects, but he chided her gently about the research. She wrote, "He pointed out to me the irrelevance of conducting surveys. He told a story to do with a man who came to inquire regarding the wonders [from] the people who had gathered, the message being that this surveyor could not learn the truth . . . in this way." The priest continued, "Medicine is split off from the spirit, but there is a lot more to medicine than science." Doctors and priests adopt each others' roles when they care for the same patient, he said, although they rarely ever see each other. "Science and medicine take us only to a certain point. Where knowledge ends, faith allows us to grasp some of the mystery." Several people stood around listening to Julia and the priest, adding their own comments, among them an elderly couple with their twin grandsons, identical boys about seven years old.

For our subjects, we were Doubting Thomases. The sociological methods study religion as an important social product without necessarily believing in the divinities as truth. For the religious, then, a statistical survey is next to meaningless, because spirituality is personal, and miracles are in the particular. It proves nothing about their existence to show that they are rare. That's the whole point.

Saddened to realize that my request had made Julia uncomfortable, I was nevertheless grateful for her efforts and her candor. It meant that the surveys could be brought to an end. Looking back now, I am also grateful to Franca Iacovetta for having insisted that we do them in the first place. The responses were indeed telling in their remarkable consistency. Although they were not the in-depth interrogation that some readers might have wanted, they revealed things that may have been obvious to the religious, but were not apparent to me. The clerics might reject the notion of surveys, but statistics have explanatory power in my world of medicine. To make the two worlds communicate, concessions had to be made in both directions. Increasingly, it was the borderland between medicine and religion that became the focus of this work. Uppermost now was the question asked at the end of Chapter 4: did medical scientists have any idea how much the saints were sharing their load? What do doctors say about miracles?

Miracle in MEDLINE: Another Survey

The surveys and the Vatican work had shown that the vast majority of miracles or acts of grace involved healing from physical illness, almost always with the additional help of medical practitioners. But most uses of the word "miracle" in our time have nothing to do with religion or the supernatural. Appearing almost daily in the media, the word means a triumph of *human* ingenuity, with the emphasis on humanity rather than divinity. It indicates achievements that confront the inexplicable or the uncontrollable to render them comprehensible and tame. In particular, popular uses of the expression "*medical* miracle" proclaim the successes of biotechnology in diagnostics and therapeutics—the opposite of the sense in which it is used by pilgrims. How exactly is the word "miracle" used in the special literature produced by doctors and scientists?

I conducted my investigation through MEDLINE—the authoritative medical science database maintained at the National Library of Medicine in Bethesda, Maryland. It now contains approximately 16 million references to articles in 5,000 journals going back as far as 1950. As of July 2010, a keyword search demonstrated that the word "miracle" was used only 805 times in the material published between 1950 and June 2010 and indexed in MEDLINE. When one considers that this database adds 40,000 to 80,000 new references every month and that it holds more than 300,000 references on the subject of "history of medicine" alone, 805 is a small number.

The vast majority (94 percent) of the 805 uses of the word "miracle" match those of the popular press. They signify marvels of *human* ingenuity. In this sense, the word "miracle" was applied to surprisingly conventional (and imperfect) drugs, such as aspirin, glucosamine, L-Dopa, insulin, and various antibiotics. It described procedures, including genetic screening, reproductive technology, and liver transplant. Some miracles were modified as "economic," "genetic," or "minor."

The use of "miracle" as an adjective was the most frequent form: miracle drug, miracle cure, miracle worker, miracle patients, miracle men, miracle babies, and one miracle heifer. More prosaic, adjectival uses of the word include proper names: for example, Miracle Village is a treatment center for addiction; and Miracle Mix is the trade name for a dental cement.

Derisive uses of the word were rare, but striking. They warned of quackery and sham science. In those instances, the word "miracle" was sometimes placed inside irony quotation marks to describe fraud, legal nightmares, mischief, mysteries, and pig food. Once it was used with a negative to detract from a successful product: would-be Lotharios were warned that "Viagra is not a miracle."

Uses of this sort have nothing to do with the miracles of the feast-day pilgrims. Only fifty-one of the 805 occurrences (or just 6 percent) were in discussions related to religion, a correspondence determined by combining the 805 results with another keyword search on "religion." Of these, many still resembled the popular media uses, despite the connection to religion. More than half (twenty-four) occurred in historical articles about saints or religious aspects of medicine's past, including Bible studies, and ancient, medieval, or early modern collections of miracle tales: four of these articles concerned Cosmas and Damian; two had been written by me. Five more debunked popular miracles by showing, for example, that stigmata were self-inflicted manifestations of hysteria, or that miraculous appearances of "blood" were actually due to overgrowth of red bacteria or phototoxic effects.[1]

Only three of the 805 articles dealt with miracles as labeled by patients: one was gently critical, although the author regretted earlier dismissiveness;[2] one analyzed skeptically;[3] and one reported on a healing with radiographic evidence that was used in the cause of Padre Pio.[4] Three articles in all of

MEDLINE addressed the kind of miracles of my pilgrims, but only the last presented the event without judgment.

Finally, and perhaps most telling, five articles warned of the dangers of expecting miracles.[5] Belief in miracles, these authors contend, leads the devout to press for ongoing, "inappropriate" care in the face of impending doom. Unnecessary and expensive treatments demanded by these patients can prolong the agony of loved ones; catering to their wishes might even be a form of discrimination against atheists. Health-care providers must be wary of such families, who should be dissuaded from their behavior by "reimagining" religious themes. The motives for these perception-altering recommendations seem diverse: one, at least, derived from aspirations for cost containment; the others sprang from professional obligations to foster realistic expectations, establish clinical authority, or maintain cultural hegemony over attitudes to death.

These five papers—all but one written by nonphysicians—were the only articles to express awareness of the prevalence and depth of spiritual hope in the health-care setting. Having made this unique observation, however, the authors urged their readers to eradicate the behavior, as if a belief in miracles was itself a disease.

To summarize the results of my "Miracle in MEDLINE" survey, in sixty years of medical publishing, only three articles—or less than 0.5 percent of the small number of articles making use of the word "miracle"—reported, without debunking, on cures that had been accepted as miracles. A far greater number are disbelieving, dismissive, or downright opposed. The point here is to emphasize the relative *lack* of attention given to religious healing in the contemporary medical imagination. This blind spot contrasts sharply with the miracles of modern pilgrims and those "official" miracles of the Vatican, which are overwhelmingly medical in nature.

MEDLINE and Prayer: Another Survey

Medical publishing is a platform for explanation. An event that lacks an explanation can enter the scientific literature only with great difficulty, usually as a case report trolling for an answer. Notwithstanding the absence of serious reporting on actual miracles, medical publishing over the last two decades has made a genuine effort to incorporate the spiritual side of patient care. The greater willingness to embrace religious topics coincides with a broadening of interest in medical humanities, especially ethics. It can be detected in recent changes to the subject classification of medical literature.

Medical subject headings (called "MeSH" headings) are designated by a team of librarians at the National Library of Medicine to make searching for articles on specific topics more efficient; they help eliminate irrelevant references that might crop up in a keyword search on MEDLINE. The precursor *Index Catalog of the Library of the Surgeon General* goes back to the late nineteenth century. It had index headings for "Religion," "Religion and Medicine," "Saints," and "Miracle." But the last word is no longer a subject heading; it and "Saints" appear to have been dropped by the time the first authoritative list of MeSH headings appeared in 1954, although "Saints" returned in 1995. Proclaiming its cultural origins in Christianity, the 1954 list also recognized, "Bible" and "Churches."[6] Several other MeSH combinations appeared by 1960 if not earlier: "Religion and Psychology," "Religion and Science," "Religion and Sex," "Religious Healings," "Prayers," and "Spiritualism." "Religion and Sociology" served briefly as a MeSH heading from 1963 to 1965. By 1966, when electronic indexing was established, headings included denominational words, such as Christianity, Hinduism, and so on. But changes in these methods of sorting were afoot. "Mental Healing," served from 1983 to 2001 only to be replaced by "Prayer Healing" and "Faith Healing," which appeared in 2002. The term, "Spirituality" also appeared in 2002.

The newness and nonspecific nature of the most recent subject headings does not imply that those topics were previously ignored. For example, the earliest reference in my "Miracle-in-MEDLINE" survey was an essay on faith healing published in 1953. Furthermore, religious doctors have published books on miraculous cures for many years, often providing medical analysis of healings found in biblical texts or in documented cures at specific shrines, such as Lourdes.[7] Those items did not turn up during the miracle search because in its vast database of peer-reviewed literature, MEDLINE does not include books or book chapters, only articles in journals.

Nevertheless, the birth date of each MeSH heading reflects a moment when the subject became of sufficient interest or importance to the medical readership to merit its own rubric. Therefore, it is fair to say that something special was happening in medical attitudes to religion and spirituality in the years leading up to 2000. This impression is further confirmed by comparing the rate of change of publishing on the topic of "Religion and Medicine" with the rate of change of all entries in MEDLINE in five-year periods (Figure 5.1). Following the first burst of data collection on all subjects in the 1960s, overall new entries in MEDLINE settled to a fairly steady rate of increase of least 10 percent or more in each five-year period. In contrast, the rate of publications on "Religion and Medicine" varied considerably through time—at least twice

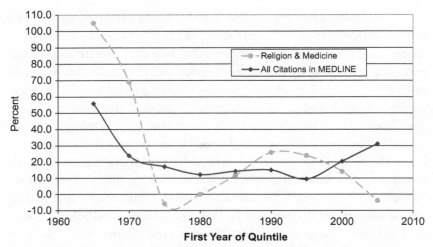

FIGURE 5.1 Percent changes in medical publishing on Religion and Medicine compared to all MEDLINE articles, 1965–2009.

declining relative to itself (falling below zero), and rising from about 1975 and for a brief period—from 1985 to 1998—actually exceeding the rate of increase of MEDLINE articles overall. Therefore, it is scarcely surprising that by 2000 new MeSH headings were needed to reflect this interest.

One factor in promoting the transient increase of interest in "Religion in Medicine" could have been the work of researchers who have tried to explore the effectiveness of prayer. The idea is not new. In 1871 a physicist, John Tyndall, suggested that the prayer healing ought to be measured against conventional care by comparing outcomes in patients occupying two different hospital wards—one prayed for, one not. His prescient suggestion for a "clinical trial" attracted many prominent thinkers and launched a controversy called "the prayer gauge debate." It has been cited as a pivotal moment in the discussion over miracles between Protestants and Catholics.[8] But it seems that no one was brave enough to actually try Tyndall's experiment for more than a century.

Hoping to bring the beneficial effects of prayer to the attention of the scientific community, researchers needed to find evidence in terms that match current notions of medical rhetoric—statistics. Ever positivistic, modern medicine sets great store by "evidence" derived from double-blind randomized controlled trials (RCTs) within the methodological trend, called Evidence-Based Medicine. "Double blinding" means that neither the patient nor the doctor knows what treatment is being used; it is intended to reduce the placebo effect, which occurs when both patient and doctor tend to perceive positive results stemming from their optimism and hopefulness. If the beneficial role of spirituality could be confirmed by well-conducted RCTs, some skeptics might be prepared to consider it. With only one exception, however, most of these publications had failed to appear in my first MEDLINE survey because these reports avoid using the word "miracle" to account for healings.[9] So I searched for these articles and explored their findings too.

Intercessory prayer (IP) entails praying for the sick by third-party strangers (or "agents") who are provided with the names and sometimes photographs of patients randomly assigned to receiving prayer or not. IP seems to have been selected as the focus of controlled trials in spirituality for several reasons: it can be documented and measured (in terms of time if not intensity); it does not harm or inconvenience sick people; and it offers the attractive possibility of randomization and double blinding—in other words, neither the doctors nor the patients themselves know who is the subject of prayer. One of the earliest such studies reported in 1988 on a trial involving nearly 400 patients admitted to a San Francisco coronary care unit: it suggested that, all other things being equal, prayer improved the course of patients whether they knew they were being prayed for or not.[10]

Over fifteen years or so, a flurry of publications reported clinical trials on IP.[11] Experimenters included Dale A. Matthews of Georgetown and Herbert Benson of Harvard. An internist, Matthews demonstrated that prayer is good for people with rheumatoid arthritis; his website is titled "The Awesome Power of God."[12] Cardiologist Benson, once labeled a "mind-body maverick" by *Science* magazine,[13] led the large STEP trial exploring the effect of prayer on 600 people undergoing coronary bypass surgery between 1998 and 2000 against an equal number of controls; it demonstrated no benefit from prayer. Indeed, those receiving prayers might have fared less well, owing to an unexplained excess of postoperative complications.[14] A Harvard-sponsored conference on "Spirituality and Healing" held in April 1999 brought 700 people of various professions to Chicago. Reflecting this trend, some medical and nursing schools began modifying their course curricula to instruct students on the importance of spirituality; not without controversy, however.[15]

Religious people were excited by the promise of these investigations for two reasons: first, medical professionals were finally taking religious practices seriously as fellow travelers in health-care provision; and second, positive results could "prove" what they already knew to be true: God exists. Authors of the STEP study were at pains to indicate that it was not designed to test the existence of God.[16] Nevertheless, some people viewed the trials in that way.

Their enthusiasm contrasts sharply with the late nineteenth-century reaction to Tyndall's call for a clinical trial.

Already by the year 2000, enough trials in IP had appeared that a team from England, led by the Reverend Leanne Roberts, reviewed the findings in the prestigious Cochrane Database of Systematic Reviews. The team used a meta-analysis, which combines a collection of clinical trials chosen on the basis of strict criteria designed to identify reliable methods. The reviewers decided that the evidence was inconclusive. Concerned that the trial method might not be right for the question, they wrote, "It could be the case that any effects are due to elements beyond present scientific understanding that will, in time, be understood. If any benefit derives from God's response to prayer it may be beyond any such trials to prove or disprove."[17]

After more than ten years of these investigations, results are mixed. Some studies suggest that prayer is beneficial (in fertility, arthritis, and anxiety). Some show that prayer has no effect, while the odd study implies that it could actually be harmful and that those who are prayed for do less well than those who are not. The *British Medical Journal* (*BMJ*) publishes humorous spoofs in its Christmas issues. In 2001 it lampooned these endeavors with a bogus report on the benefits of *retroactive* intercessory prayer for people who were already dead of sepsis.[18] The article occasioned a bouquet of witty letters to the editor, printed the following April. But by December 2009, a team in Denmark noticed that, in twelve of thirty-six subsequent citations, the *BMJ*'s fake article had been accepted at face value as serious research. The Danish team then targeted the sanctimonious aspects of Evidence-Based Medicine, by documenting a new source of scientific bias: the Serious Idiopathic Loss of Ludic ironY (or SILLY) bias.[19]

Roberts's team updated their 2000 Cochrane review twice. First, in 2007, the reviewers concluded that, although most data were "equivocal," the evidence was "interesting enough to justify further study into the human aspects of the effects of prayer." But they were attacked by the Danish group (of the SILLY bias) for the "unsound and unhelpful" conclusions that failed to live up to the high standards of Cochrane reviews. Possibly remembering the *BMJ* of Christmas 2001, the Danes closed their rout with this remark: "the author assured us that the review was not a joke, which we had hoped it was."[20]

The second Cochrane update by Roberts's team came soon after, in 2009, and ended with a reversal: "These findings are equivocal and, although some of the results of individual studies suggest a positive effect of intercessory prayer, the majority do not and the evidence does not support a recommendation either in favor or against the use of intercessory prayer. We are not convinced that further trials of this intervention should be undertaken and would prefer to see any resources available for such a trial used to investigate other questions in health care."[21] The full effects of this powerful statement on subsequent research into IP are yet to be revealed; however, in the last ten years, the rate of medical publishing on religion relative to all other medical publication has plummeted (Figure 5.1).

In the meantime, others expressed strong reservations about the logistics and the ethics of such work. Prayer is not the same as a drug: the vast theoretical disjunction—between believers who pray and the medical caregivers who do not—renders the exercise meaningless.[22] One writer pointed out that the studies are ethically problematic for true believers who serve as agents of prayers: they cannot live up to their own principles without subverting the investigation by praying for members of a designated control group who ought to receive no prayers.[23] An Australian observer (and self-avowed atheist) found that researchers exploring IP through trials had ignored the "gold-standard" basics of ethics in terms of patient confidentiality, standards of care, and informed consent. Furthermore, he argued, they were guilty of having assumed that prayer posed no safety risks to its subjects; therefore, he contended, applying the results would be ethically problematic.[24] Another well-known atheist decried the experiments as "infantile theology"; however, he appeared to acknowledge a cultural role for religion and expressed a desire for more and better experiments: "It would be a mistake to suppose that the nonexistence of an intercessory-prayer benefit would show that prayer is a useless practice. There are subtler benefits to be evaluated—but they do need to be identified."[25] His more militant colleague heaped several pages of vitriol on the STEP study, calling it a "pathetic" and "barmy exercise."[26] Fully confirming the entrenched gulf between medical science and religion and citing their own views as dominant, another pair of critics asserted that "these studies claim findings incompatible with current views of the physical universe and consciousness," adding that they "should not be conducted."[27] Far be it from science to explore new views of the universe.

Most damaging of all, a report on spirituality in the medical care of the seriously ill suggests that intercessory prayer may be the least important of such practices by those who set any store by them.[28]

After their heady beginning, the clinical trials on spirituality seem to have missed the boat; they signify nothing. Julia's priest in Toronto could have predicted that, and he would not have been the least bit deflected from his faith.

More Feasts: Brooklyn and Conshohocken, PA

Stopping the surveys had been liberating. We could now visit feast-day events simply to observe, enjoy, and learn, without having to question strangers. With his verve and curiosity, Bert Hansen was ever vigilant for new possibilities. Aware that the feast for the santi medici might be nothing more than another transplanted Italian celebration, we wanted to sample Italian feste that were focused on other saints. So it was that Bert took us to the "dance of the *giglio*" in Brooklyn's Williamsburg neighborhood in July 2003. The *nec plus ultra* of Italian feasts, this twelve-day extravaganza was featured in Tony DeNonno's documentary, "Heaven Touches Brooklyn in July" (2001). Its origin is definitely religious, honoring San Paolino, an early fifth-century bishop who sacrificed his freedom for that of his flock in Nola, southern Italy. But the rite of veneration had become something else entirely.[29]

In honor of San Paolino, 125 American men lift a platform that holds a five-story, five-ton, lily-encrusted, papier-maché pillar, a fifteen-piece brass band and a priest (Figure 5.2). With liftoff, they "dance" the towering ensemble through the streets in time to folk music. A giant ship also raised on a dais participates in this muscular retelling. The annual event is in direct

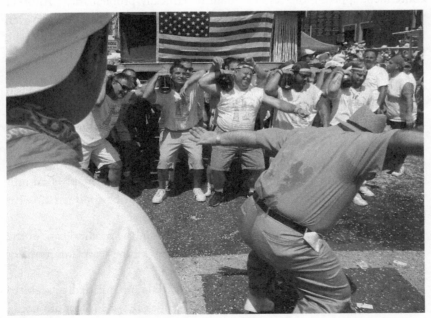

FIGURE 5.2 Dance of the Giglio, capo and lifters, Williamsburg, Brooklyn, NY, 2003. Photo by Robert David Wolfe.

sympathy with the original in Nola, where not one but eight pillars are involved. We were amazed at the energy, power, and preparation involved in creating this celebration—and we were nearly run over when we accidentally got trapped between the crowd and the swaying ship. Leaving its religious connections aside, the *giglio* did not seem to be medical at all.

Then in 2005, we found the website of Saints Cosmas and Damian Church, Conshohocken, Pennsylvania. Like the feast in Utica, it had been established in 1912 by Italian immigrants; however, they had come from Isernia to work in the Philadelphia-area factories. Parish services were held in the large basement foundation from 1926, and later in the Romanesque stone church above, the construction of which began in 1951. The ceiling is entirely covered in paintings of Jesus, Mary, and various saints, by parishioner Emmanuel Utti, as the website says, "a la the Sistine chapel in Rome." Begun in the 1950s, the ceiling was restored by the artist and his son in 2002. References to familiar images abound: Utti's *pietà* was based on Michelangelo's, while his Cosmas and Damian had been inspired by the 1950s "Great Moments" series of Robert Thom, first commissioned and mass-produced by Parke-Davis drug company for advertising displays in pharmacy windows (Figure 5.3). The latter was another surprising collision of research projects, as

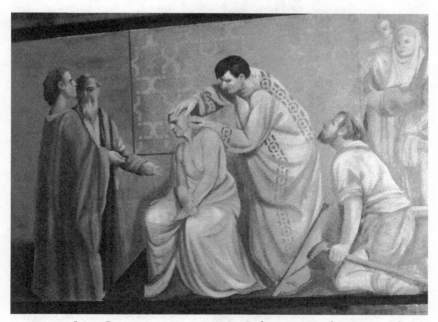

FIGURE 5.3 Saint Cosmas treating a patient. Ceiling painting by Emmanuel Utti, Conshocken, PA, circa 1960.

I had written on the popularity and purpose of the "Great Moments" paintings a few years earlier.[30] Despite the enormous success and wide distribution
of that commercial art series, never did I imagine it would have influenced
religious art.

Bert and I planned to drive to Conshohocken from Manhattan, but the
trains had suffered a massive power outage and swarms of thwarted passen-
gers crammed the car rental agency. By the time we arrived later that day, a
crowd of several hundred had already assembled (Figure 5.4). This ninety-first
feast followed the usual pattern: three days of masses in honor of the saints, a
Saturday night vigil, and a Sunday mass and daytime procession, followed by
a healing service that ended with hands-on blessings at the altar rail. A street
market, booths, and amusement rides enliven the celebration to the benefit of
the school.

The Italian roots of the founders were featured here too. But we soon
noticed that many of these pilgrims were not of Italian origin. They were African American and they seemed to be speaking French—until we realized it
was Creole. These were Haitian immigrants, just like the women whom Julia

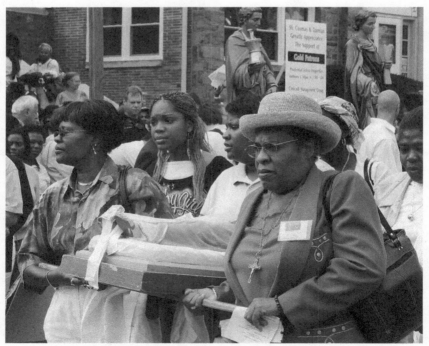

FIGURE 5.4 Procession leaving church, Conshohocken, PA, 2005. Photo by Bert Hansen.

had encountered in Cambridge—but in far greater numbers. At the time, it was a relief not to have to conduct any interviews. I was going to phone the deacon when I got home and could ask about the pilgrims later. We admired the church, followed the procession, watched the services, took pictures, and indulged in delicious focaccia and cannoli. The healing service exuded an electric atmosphere as the church was packed with chanting worshippers, waving both arms high in praise. Following the ceremonies, people lingered in mellow conviviality. In the church basement, a stout man burst into an operatic aria in a splendid tenor, but he was ignored.

Later, I learned that Robert Orsi had spotted and analyzed Haitian interest in Italian street feste in Harlem.[31] But the Conshohocken organizers did not know where their Haitian worshippers had come from. They gave me the name of Father Albert Gardy, a Haitian-born priest in nearby Philadelphia; he remembered them vividly, but they were not from his parish. He gave me the name of Mary Moïse, one of his parishioners who organized cultural events. She knew some first names but no surnames, and she was not sure where they lived. She supposed, however, that Cosmas and Damian were known and loved in Haiti. I regretted stopping the surveys.

In the fall of 2010, I was planning to be at the Toronto feast, but I also wanted to visit Conshohocken again—the same old problem of trying to be in two places at once. Canadian Rachel Elder, finishing her history doctorate at University of Pennsylvania, kindly volunteered to be my research-assistant-for-a-day. She went back to Conshohocken with the revived "survey instrument" and the permission of the church. Rachel found that about half the pilgrims were of Italian origin, and the other half had indeed come from Haiti; the latter group lived mostly in Brooklyn, although she met one from Montreal. They came on busses that had been booked by touring groups and pilgrimage organizations rather than any parish.

Rachel's findings mirrored those of the earlier surveys. The twin-aspect was important to more than half; the doctor-aspect was equally important, especially to those with nurses and doctors in the family. And again, more than half (64 percent) claimed to know of miracles, with most of the miracles described being healings. A few people recognized their successful immigration to the United States as a divine miracle. Many of the Haitian Americans had been on pilgrimages to other centers: the shrines of Frances Cabrini, Notre Dame de Salette, St. Jude, and in Quebec, Ste. Anne de Beaupré and Notre Dame du Cap. One eighty-year-old Haitian woman who had been in the United States since 1969 claimed to have been to Conshohocken more than twenty-five times. As to whether Cosmas and

Damian had been important back in Haiti or discovered in the United States, we obtained conflicting answers and thus the matter was not clear.

Saints Cosmas and Damian of Haiti?

Scholars have been active on this topic for at least two decades. Cosmas and Damian were connected symbiotically—or "syncretized"—to the twin gods of African traditional religions, by the Yoruba in what is now Nigeria and Ghana and by the Fon in Benin. They have become the Marassa of Vodou or the Ibeji (also Ibeye) of Santería in Caribbean countries and Brazil. These deities are members of the lwas, who are the Haitian traditional spirits.[32] In Africa and Haiti, the twins are not doctors but mischievous children; they are said to become jealous, even vindictive, if not given their due. But as Marilyn Houlberg had suggested, they too were linked to medicine even in Africa, because of the vulnerability of children to illness and their need for special care.[33] The Marassa know healing plants and are also invoked for problems of property, justice, and marriage. Some see them as homosexual partners, emblematic of certain features of Vodou that drew opprobrium from Christian authorities. Johan Wedel conducted a survey on the nature of appeals to the traditional twins in Cuba and found that fully half are for illness, with 90 percent of the responses including recommendations to consult an ordinary physician.[34]

Apparently Cosmas and Damian enjoy a following in Haiti. But now it is easier to find information on their role within African traditions in that country rather than within the Catholic Church. According to Patrick Bellegarde-Smith the distance between the medical saints and the twin lwas has grown wider as the ruthless persecution of African rituals declined.[35] Nevertheless, photographs of Vodou altars sometimes display a familiar lithograph of the santi medici—in their youthful, beardless form. In other words, the image that often appears on Roman Catholic prayer cards has been embraced and transformed in Haitian folk art.[36] Heike Drotbohm, who studies the large Haitian community in Montreal, claims that the private shrine of "every female Vodouisant has a symbol of the Marassa who are represented by the Catholic Saints, St. Cosmas and St. Damian"[37] (Figure 5.5). The santi medici have also been spotted on Vodou altars in Brooklyn.[38] In Haiti, at La Plaine Peristil, north of Port-au-Prince, photographer Chantal Regnault captured a banner of the Haitian Marassa with evident cultural debt to the saints (Figure 5.6). At the time of writing and for the preceding two years, a Google image search on "Marassa" produced a picture of Cosmas and Damian.

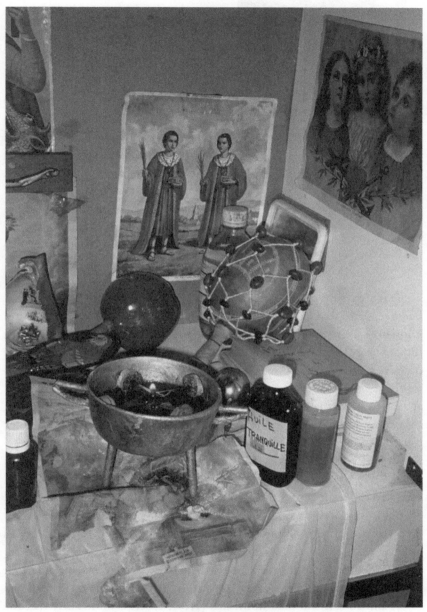

FIGURE 5.5 Cosmas and Damian as Marassa on a vodou shrine in Montreal, 2002. Photo courtesy of Heike Drotbohm.

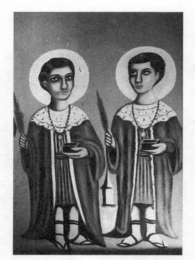

FIGURE 5.6 Marassa based on Cosmas and Damian, Haiti, 1993. Photo by Chantal Regnault.

Some observers virtually "accuse" the church of having deliberately encouraged this slippage between Catholic saints and the traditional lwas—all the better to evangelize and control natives and slaves. For example, in 1965, Roger Bastide wrote: "sociologically the Church well understood [the appeal to archetypes], for it tried to sublimate and spiritualize the beliefs of the enslaved Africans departing from their animism, to find substitutes that would allow education of religious sentiment without doing violence [*viol*] to souls."[39] In other words, allowing Cosmas and Damian to stand in for the Marassa was a way of "selling" Christianity to the slaves.

This argument strongly resembles the one, discussed in Chapter 2, that had been used to explain the relationship of the santi medici to the pagan Dioscuri—a promotion maneuver nearly two thousand years old. But it implies that the worshippers had no role at all in the decision to recognize divinities. Granted, the Caribbean "converts" were slaves; yet spiritual commitment might have been their only remaining freedom. Assigning more agency to slaves than did Bastide, Laennec Hurbon goes so far as to suggest that the slaves and natives deliberately took Christian saints as foils for hiding their own deities, allowing their traditions to survive and develop.[40] Oppressed by Christians, then, practitioners of Vodou hid their beliefs behind select Christian forms, just as the oppressed early Christians had appealed to pagan deities and concealed their rituals in the catacombs.

But it is projecting a great deal of awareness on to the early modern colonizers to assert that they understood enough of African or Native traditions to be able to identify those saints that would best appeal as homologues for Indians or slaves. Could they have had this knowledge by the time that Cosmas and Damian were chosen as patrons for the earliest church in Brazil (1535) and an early hospital in Mexico (1539)? It seems more likely that the medical saints were chosen by religious colonizers either for their special medical functions or out of nostalgia for the patrons of home. Similarly, it demands too much knowledge of Catholicism in the oppressed, illiterate slaves to suggest that they knew which saints to "hide" behind. For them, the

saints and the lwas merged perfectly. They were two versions of the same transcendent essence, in much the same way that Jehovah, Allah, and God are
one. As political and social pressures caused people to conspicuously turn
away from Vodou, some suggest that Protestantism was a safer choice because
the Roman Catholic saints could be suspected substitutes for the lwas.[41]
Others reported conversions from Vodou to Protestantism (not Catholicism)
following cures effected by modern medicine.[42]

For these reasons, some scholars reject the term, "syncretism," in favor of
words such as "fusion" or "symbiosis."[43] The two traditions influenced each
other: the feasts of the Marassa or the Ibeye coincide with that of the santi
medici. In some places, the Christian Cosmas and Damian assume the child
identity and function of the Marassa—or vice versa. Thus, on September 27,
especially in Rio de Janeiro, bags of candy, stamped with the saints' images, are
given to the Roman Catholic children of Brazil to protect them in the coming
year.[44] And on that same day, Haitian immigrants come to worship at American Catholic shrines built by immigrants from Italy. Elsewhere, the childhood
connection has allowed Cosmas and Damian feasts to shift from September
to Christmas.[45] In these practices, it seems African traditions have influenced
Christianity.

The Haitian pilgrims at the Cosmas and Damian feast in Conshohocken
described themselves as good Catholics, not followers of Vodou; sometimes
they volunteered their home parishes. Indeed, as sociologist Margarita
Mooney observed, the scholarly attention to Vodou is disproportionate to its
apparent role in Haiti; more than 60 percent of Haitians identify as Catholics, while only 11 percent claim to follow Vodou.[46] The Conshohocken pilgrims may never have heard of the Marassa, but it is also not clear that they
knew of Cosmas and Damian before coming to the United States. To the
best of my knowledge, no Catholic churches in Haiti are under the patronage
of Cosmas and Damian. Although many pilgrims of Haitian origin recall
similar feast-day celebrations, none could identify any particular veneration
of the twin doctors in that country.

Born in Jacmel, Haiti, pilgrim Yolette Toussaint told us that journeying is
how she prays, and it is how many Haitian people pray. Back home, she used to
visit Notre Dame de la Charité at Carrefour Feuilles, near Port-au-Prince. One
day in 1980, while she lay on the floor, hands outstretched and lost in prayer, she
had a vision of a man wearing a long, green robe and holding a staff; he handed
her a little book and she remembers distinctly that it was a passport. Later,
Yolette told her mother: "I'm gonna go somewhere, I don't know where, but
I'm goin'." Her mother was amused, but Yolette was on her way to New York

within the year. In the United States, she searched for a long time to find a way to go on pilgrimages. "My pilgriming is my prayer," she said. This yearning was satisfied when the husband of her babysitter led her to one of the Haitian organizations that specialize in religious travel; the original organizer has long since died. Yolette has been to Conshohocken at least three times, not because of the saints, but because the Italian feast is a pretext for pilgrimage. Through the journey she learned to venerate the twin doctors and their works.[47]

The importance of pilgrimages in Haitian spirituality of all denominations has not escaped the notice of scholars. Some Haitians describe life itself as a journey or a pilgrimage of suffering.[48] It would be tempting to attribute this interest in traveling prayer to the Christianization of the island by Iberian missionaries who sojourned there. But scholar Terry Rey suggests, instead, that its ethnic origins derive from an older Christian impulse stemming from medieval customs and hailing from the Congo in Central Africa rather than West Africa; he contends that some slaves brought it with them from Africa.[49] These intriguing arguments draw upon several classic sites of veneration in Haiti, such as Carrefour Feuilles and Saut d'Eau (Sodo), to show that the pilgrimage phenomenon transcends religious boundaries. Rey's observations back up the story told by Yolette Toussaint. She found Cosmas and Damian because she needed a journey in order to pray.

The success of Cosmas and Damian with converts to Christianity from devotees of other twins gods, either in pagan antiquity or from modern West Africa, invokes the psychological—rather than sociological or genealogical—explanation for their durability. As explained in Chapter 2, this theory of universal Dioscurism holds that holy twins are discovered and rediscovered through the permanence and significance of dual archetypes in the human mind: the super vitality of double birth and the natural harmony of primal opposites, uniting earth and sky, day and night, disease and health, life and death. Saints Cosmas and Damian were available in the New World because European clerics delivered them, thinking that they were appropriate. They stayed and flourished because they made sense to the people whom they served—because they were twins, or because they were doctors, or because they were celebrated with feasts and travel.

Tangled Threads

The conversations with Haitians suggested that my project had been a pilgrimage too: physical travel to the sites of veneration in the New and Old Worlds; and virtual mind travel that moved a long way from the positivistic orientation of my medical studies. My pilgrimage may not have been a prayer to a deity, but it was nevertheless an act of devotion to the beauty and power of inquiry.

The quest had endured for so long that key players began to disappear. In Howard Beach, Father Evans and Joe DeCandia have both died; however, the energetic veneration that they founded carries on without them, focusing now on support for research into childhood diabetes. Ersilia Jannetta has also passed away, but the statues that she brought to Toronto still make their annual September pilgrimage through the neighborhood streets, while the feast-day mass continues to pack the church whether or not the congregation has heard of her pivotal role.

Sadly, Pierre Julien died in 2007, and his vast Cosmas and Damien collection was dispersed. The distinguished New York collector and historian William (Bill) Helfand rescued many of the prints and engravings. Bill generously invited us to his Manhattan apartment to see the acquisitions that were being carefully identified and cataloged with the help of students. I inherited several prints and a cluster of Catalan *goigs* from 1881 to 1982—each one a reminder that every site must have its own peculiar reason for establishing a feast; each one a reminder that my study had merely scratched the surface of a labyrinthine array of devotions to the santi medici (Figure 5.7).[50]

In 2010 both the American Association for the History of Medicine and the American Osler Society met in Rochester, Minnesota, home of the Mayo Clinic. The turnout was enormous because the historians of medicine were eager to see and learn more about the legendary medical center. Bert Hansen and I were among them.

This highly respected nonprofit organization was founded by physician William W. Mayo and his two doctor sons: William J. (Will) and Charles Mayo (Figure 5.8). A master narrative tells how in 1883 a disastrous tornado ravaged the community. Mother Alfred Moes, head of the local teaching order of Franciscan nuns, offered to raise funds to build a hospital, provided that the elder Mayo would serve as its doctor. Saint Marys Hospital was the result. The sons trained in medicine with a special interest in surgery and returned to Rochester. Their skill was legendary, the postoperative results enviable, and other doctors came from far and wide to observe and work. One secret to their immense success was the formation of a group practice from as early as 1892; another was the clever decision to create a foundation so that succession, money, and ownership were never in question. They died within a few weeks of each other in 1939, but their "clinic" simply carried on to ever greater achievement: more facilities, bigger buildings, and the best technology.

GOIGS EN LLOANÇA DELS GLORIOSOS METGES I MARTIRS SANT COSME I SANT DAMIA

VENERATS A LA SANTA ESGLESIA CATEDRAL BASILICA DE BARCELONA

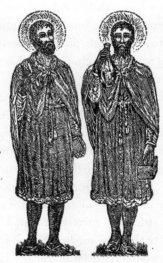

PUIX per vostra santa mà,
 Déu ens mostra sa clemència,
Sant Cosme i Sant Damià,
 féu-nos lleu tota dolència.
De l'Aràbia en gran ciutat
naixeu, oh preclars germans!
que entre mig de tants pagans,
el ver Déu sempre heu buscat.
Ja majors vau professar
del guarir, l'alta ciència.
 Sant...
Seguint sempre la virtut
ennoblíreu vostres cors,
i cercant cèlics tresors
mirant la Creu heu viscut.
Per això el Cel mostrà
vers tots dos sa preferència.
 Sant...
Jutjats per Lísies en sou
i acusats de cristians,
fins que ben lligats de mans
vostra condemna es conclou.
Enfrontats amb el tirà
sou tractats amb violència.
 Sant...
En tal guisa condemnats
vau ésser gitats al fons
de la mar, mostrant-vos bons
cristians, mes sou salvats.
De la mort us deslliurà
la Divina Omnipotència.
 Sant...

Llavors sou llançats al foc,
mes el braç omnipotent
allunya aquell flam ardent
que no us crema molt ni poc.
Inútil doncs va restar
del tirà la greu sentència.
 Sant...
Lísies ja tot furiós,
va manar que degollats
fóssiu; per això exaltats
sou al Cel amb cant gojós.
Vostra fe us va enlairar
a la més alta excel·lència.
 Sant...
Els miracles que haveu fet
no tenen compte ni fi;
prou pot dir-se que a desdir
vostra amor regna a pleret.
Conhort cert podrà trobar
qui us pregui amb diligència.
 Sant...
Barcelona us ha mostrat
devoció sempre esplendent,
puix en cas de sofriment
sou remei ben comprovat.
Per això volem pregar
vostre ajut amb reverència.
 Sant...
Puix per vostra santa mà,
Déu ens mostra sa clemència:
Sant Cosme i Sant Damià,
féu-nos lleu tota dolència.

AQUESTA EDICIO VA ESSER patrocinada per En Joan Subirachs i Farràs de Barcelona, col·leccionista de goigs, i s'estampà en recordança de la seva Exposició de 122 goigs dels gloriosos màrtirs Sant Cosme i Sant Damià, celebrada al noble edifici que el Gremi entre Tenders-Revenedors posseeix a la Plaça del Pi de la Ciutat Comtal. L'Exposició restà oberta al públic del 20 al 30 d'octubre del 1961. En l'acte inaugural pronuncià una notable conferència el Doctor A. Castillo de Lucas, de Madrid.

℣. Lætámini in Dómino, et exultáti justi. ℟. Et gloriámini omnes recti corde.

OREMUS

PRÆSTA, quaésumus, omnípotens Deus: ut, qui sanctórum Mártyrum tuórum Cosmæ et Damiáni natalítia cólimus, a cunctis malis imminéntibus, eórum intercessiónibus, liberémur. Per Christum Dóminum nostrum.
 ℟. Amen.

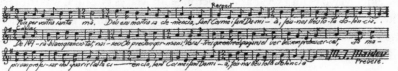

Text antic anònim, revisat per R. Vives i Sabaté autor de les xilografies. Música de Mn. Josep Maideu i Auguet, Prev.
Amb llicència eclesiàstica. Any MCMLXI.

R.V.S.

FIGURE 5.7 Catalan goigs in honor of the glorious doctors and martyrs, with poetry and music. A special edition for an exhibit, Barcelona, Spain, 1961. Gift of William Helfand.

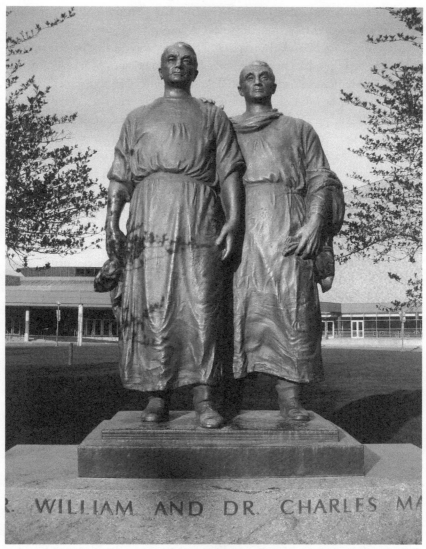

FIGURE 5.8 Statues of William and Charles Mayo, brothers and physicians, Rochester, MN, 2010.

Several statues of the brothers, their father, and Mother Moes grace the city. An excellent museum preserves their legacy—shrinelike—around the original offices in the Plummer building, Saint Marys Hospital, and the new Gonda building. Bert and I visited these places avidly, and we also spent time in the hospital chapel. Letters from political leaders, royalty, grateful patients,

Nobel laureates, and other famous scientists hang on the walls with reconstructed images of their work. Devotion, relics, and ex-votos.

Mayo cardiologist and historian Dr. Bruce Fye was hosting both meetings,
as he wrapped up his term at the helm of the American Association for the
History of Medicine. His Presidential Address derived from his forthcoming
history of the Mayo Clinic; he argues convincingly that the center had created a model for postgraduate training in all specialties. For the cover of the
American Osler Society program, Bruce and his colleagues selected a color
lithograph of Saints Cosmas and Damian that William Osler had picked up
"in the Mother Church" of the medical saints in Rome in 1906 and sent to
Will Mayo in 1915 (Figure 5.9). In the accompanying letter, Osler wrote that
he "was delighted to find wrapped in a parcel among the precious relics the
very instruments with which in the 3rd century A.D. these famous surgeons
had performed the transplantation of the thigh operation—and successfully,
too—antedating [Alexis] Carrel about 1700 years. It is a cheap print as you
see but the merit of it is that it comes direct from the shrine of the saints."
Later, in reassuring a colleague about to undergo surgery, he again told the
story of his trip to Rome "where [he] burnt a candle—a small one—for [his]
surgical colleagues," calling Will Mayo, "The American St. Cosmas."[51]

Osler identified some undeniable parallels in the life work of the two pairs
of brother doctors. But—notwithstanding their debt to the Franciscan
nuns—the Mayo family was not Roman Catholic, William senior came from
England, and his sons were not twins. They belonged to a Protestant church,
but often they were too busy on Sunday mornings to attend to services. If
medicine was not their religion, it had certainly become a religion for many
people in their sphere.

Having just invested months in unraveling the connection of the saints to
the African religious traditions of the New World, I was charmed. The project
now garnered celebrity endorsements from Bruce Fye and from the secular,
medical saints William Osler and the brothers Mayo. And it found yet another startling juxtaposition: Catholic saints recognized and remembered, if
not venerated, in a nonprofit, medical mecca founded by Protestant brothers
who rarely went to church.

Back to Rome

"That wall was built in 77," Brother Mark McBride said with a big smile. We
were sitting in the office of the Basilica of Saints Cosmas and Damian, where
a thoughtful plasterer had embellished the ancient office wall with a few

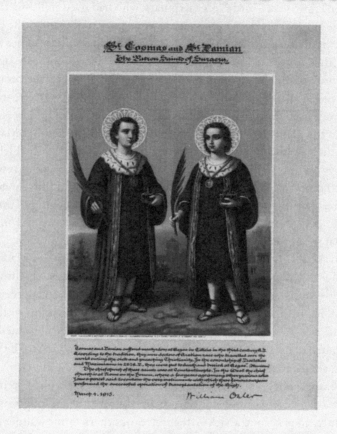

FIGURE 5.9 Cover of the 2010 program for the American Osler Society meeting at the Mayo Clinic with the image of Saints Cosmas and Damian sent to the Mayo brothers by William Osler. Use of the image of the lithograph of St. Cosmas and St. Damian by the American Osler Society courtesy of Mayo Foundation for Medical Education and Research, Mayo Historical Collection.

smooth holes offering glimpses of the massive original stones. "The Map of Rome used to hang just outside." Invited to Italy to speak about the *Medical Miracles* book in June 2010, I could not resist another visit to the basilica of the santi medici in Rome, hoping to learn the place of scientific medicine in its yearly cycle. We were lucky to meet with the American-born friar, a member of the Franciscan Third Order Regulars, who had lived in Rome for three years. The Franciscans occupy the adjoining convent and manage the basilica, and they have done so since the 1500s and its days as an insalubrious swamp. Around that time, the impoverished order was unceremoniously uprooted from a more desirable site near the Piazza Farnese. It fell to the brothers to manage the basilica, its garden, pastures, and hospice; they still have the cattle brands once used for marking animals in the Campo Vaccino. They also ministered to the many people living in the vicinity, until, as Brother Mark said, "we lost the neighborhood." He was referring to the excavations, which began tentatively in the eighteenth century, increasing into the nineteenth and twentieth centuries, and ending with Benito Mussolini's "improvement plan," which created the grandiose Via dei Fori Imperiali by bulldozing all the dwellings and many antiquities. Archeologists are back, but no one else now lives along that great, sterile street.

With a background in mathematics and finance, Brother Mark's chief function is to preside over the books of his order in its missions throughout the world—all in honor of St. Francis, whom we'd come to appreciate way back in Chapter 1. But Brother Mark feels a powerful devotion to the twin saints too, and he loves their basilica—a gathering place, he reminded us. He spends much of his free time on evenings and weekends talking to the visitors, pilgrims, and tourists.

The basilica celebrates a Triduum leading up to the feast on September 26, but none of the events are specifically medical. Nevertheless, pilgrims appear "constantly" to pray for the sick—themselves or others. Some wander into the sanctuary with no idea why they came. Brother Mark often discovers that they are ailing, or worried about someone else. He explains as much about the history and the saints as they want to hear, but he calmly accepts their atheism or their greater interest in the architecture, art, mosaics, and the nearby forum, supplying whatever information he can.

Brother Mark knew of the links to the ancient temple of Castor and Pollux and the Fountain of Juturna, just a stone's throw away—and it did not bother him in the slightest if the veneration of the saints at this site was a descendent of pagan tradition. He was excited by the notion that the Greek physician Galen may have taught medicine at the door to the basilica, because one of the second-century functions of the building had been as a library. The pharmacy guild still resides next door in the San Lorenzo in Miranda Church, itself occupying the former Roman temple to Faustina and Antoninus (Figure 2.6). Once a year representatives of the basilica of the santi medici participate in the solemn ceremony to accept new pharmacists, just as they have done since 1799. Brother Mark happily pointed out the linguistic slippage that caused the ancient image above the altar to shift in meaning from "greeting" to "health." This Madonna della Salute once spoke aloud to chide Pope Gregory the Great, who had become too busy to bother "saluting" her anymore; in the ambiance of the basilica, the miraculous image soon was known as the Madonna of Health (also *salute*). Women pray to her hoping for children. He also knew of the feast-day celebrations to the santi medici in America, and the child-focused devotion in Brazil, where, he said, "It's huge!" Organizers of these New World events are frequent visitors to the basilica.

"We still get requests for incubation," the friar said. "People ask if they can sleep in the church." Shortly after he arrived in Rome, a woman came to inquire if she could spend the night in the sanctuary. At first, he thought her question extremely odd, but it prompted him to learn more about that ancient method of treatment and its connection to the basilica. After all, this was the place where the saints were said to have worked their transplantation miracle of the black leg. Now he understands and would accommodate such requests if possible, although they are not actively advertised. Security is an issue and thefts have happened—for example the Madonna's golden crown was stolen. The monks are also concerned about serving the very sick during the night. Catering to these desires, a woman in Rome named Barbara organizes bus trips to a Cosmas and Damian shrine somewhere in the south—perhaps it is Riace—where facilities are set up for incubation.

"In a sense we are the 'mother church' of the medical saints," Brother Mark said, like Osler before him. As a result, he thinks that the basilica could do more specifically in terms of healing. It is a great favorite for weddings, but Brother Mark would like to see more done for sick people and for physicians. He mentioned healing masses as one possibility to help medicine find its way.

Brother Mark was organizing a day-long conference on medicine and religion with collaborators from the Mayo Clinic where I had been only a few weeks earlier. He hoped it would be opened with a short discourse on Galen by philosophy professor Giulia Lombardi of the Angelicum, the Pontifical University of Saint Thomas Aquinas in Rome. Without knowing of William Osler's gift of the poster, he had already identified parallels in the Mayo

Clinic's history with the twin saints—brother healers, good medicine, selfless service, and a nonprofit structure. The connection struck him as obvious. He said that Will and Charlie Mayo had visited the basilica.

I asked if he knew of the veneration in Haiti and the syncretizing with Vodou lwas. He did not, but it wouldn't surprise or upset him at all. "Ministry poses an opportunity." The details of people's stories, the gestures of invocation matter little. In thinking about "how to appeal to people with little education," insisting dogmatically on only one view is not helpful. "At the core is a message of spirituality." It is each person's "individual quest to figure out what is beyond." Guides come in different forms—as "companions on our journey of life; they can be living or dead." Ritual practice and tradition all have their place as an accompaniment for medicine on the spirit-led human adventure. "There's an anarchist in all of us," he said with a grin. If the saints match the African lwas, or the brothers Mayo, then on some level, that is exactly who they are. "It is a devotion that cannot be stamped out. Nationalism might be a starting point, but devotion is really about individual minds and hearts." Enacting faith is a therapeutic ritual in itself.

Rituals in medical practice are legion, but they are rarely commented upon in the literature. A classic article from 1959 poked anthropological fun at many of the tropes of our health behaviors; it is still cited.[52] People involved in nursing and palliative care seem to have paid the most attention to the benefits of ritual, not only for patients but also for caregivers; they rightly identify its presence in a variety of gestures, from anointing patients with alcohol swabs, to the donning of white robes, to the evening tea break and the "handing over" report.[53] The odd observer condemns ritual as a pernicious waste of time and money and recommends that it be ferreted out in a seek-and-destroy operation.[54] But others, ranging from surgeons to hospital administrators, accept its inevitability and utility.[55] Practicing medicine resembles the doing of religion in more ways than we generally admit.

Brother Mark joined us for a delightful lunch al fresco at the residence of Anne Leahy, Canadian ambassador to the Holy See and our old friend from Paris days. She had invited a group of journalists and clerics who were working on causes for Canadian saints, and we were joined by Sister Mary Casey, postulator for the cause of Mother Mary MacKillop. In October 2010 Mother Mary would become Australia's first saint on the same day as Frère André would become Canada's second saint. Here we were, back in the same Roman house by the San Sebastiano gate where twenty years earlier we had celebrated the first Canadian-born saint, Marguerite d'Youville. Talk round the table was of miracles: those from ongoing causes, the one I had witnessed, those I could summarize from my book, and the recently revealed healing of an Australian woman with metastatic lung cancer, which she had ascribed to Mother Mary MacKillop. Frère André was a thaumaturge in his life and he is said to have interceded many times after his death, but the miracle used for his canonization had yet to be revealed.

Brother Mark listened quietly and with interest, but Cosmas and Damian had never been subjected to these arduous proofs. They became saints long before the rules had been laid down, and, although they were healers in life and beyond too, their claim to sanctity was martyrdom. They were saints not only because of how they lived, but especially because of how and why they had died. More than medicine, then, death was a silent actor in this piece. Death demanded more attention.

THESE TRAVELS HAD revived the psychological theory to explain the reason for Cosmas and Damian in Toronto. The slippage between the Christian twins and the Haitian Marassa, or the secular Mayo heroes, provided surprising evidence for their connection to the ancient Dioscuri and other more distant twin healers—relationships that had nothing to do with Italian nationalism or nostalgia for homeland—relationships that might speak of an eternal, innate proclivity to find healers in twins. The surveys and the Vatican research had demonstrated the robust interconnectedness of illness, healing, medicine, and religion, but medical sources are mostly silent on the matter, despite honest attempts to bring spirituality into discussions of health care.

Miracles—official and unofficial—do not seem to happen without scientific medicine. But most doctors seem utterly unaware of the importance of their own discipline in the lived experience of faith. That gap still needs to be explained.

6

Conclusion

HOME TO THE CLINIC

*We pretend that modern medicine is a rational science, all
facts, no nonsense, and just what it seems. But we have only
to tap its glossy veneer for it to split wide open, and reveal to
us its roots and foundations, its old dark heart of meta-
physics, mysticism, magic, and myth.*
—OLIVER SACKS, *Awakenings, 1973, Prologue, 28*

SO NOW AFTER all these travels, we have two contradictory, if not mutually
exclusive, observations. Based on the surveys of the scientific literature, discussed in the previous chapter, medical professionals largely ignore miracles,
and sometimes try to dissuade people from believing in them. They are also
uncomfortable with spirituality at the bedside, although they try hard to
respect it. But for the feast-day pilgrims, miracles are plausible occurrences
that usually entail *physical* cures, enacted through (or in spite of) a conventional caregiver, a physician, or a surgeon. The same is true for those "official"
miracles in the Vatican archives investigated by the church. I am far from
being the first to have noticed this predominance of healings and medicine in
the range of miracles that extend beyond the boundaries to Protestantism and
to other religions.[1]

Whether or not clinical trials demonstrate statistical benefits, those who
pray are convinced of the importance of the saints—not only for the connections to faith, cultural roots, and local traditions, but also for their active
and ongoing participation in the comfort and care of the sick. Positive
results in trials are almost beside the point. Yet physicians do not write
about it.

Most doctors would admit that they cannot explain everything—*yet*. A
special "scientific" vocabulary has been developed to accommodate that reality
with words like "spontaneous," "idiopathic," "essential," and "placebo." Those

words appear with great frequency in the literature, in contrast to words that are spiritually charged—miracle, prayer, faith. Like medical language, the *methods* of science also permit ignoring: no experiment can be designed to falsify supernatural intervention.[2] The handful of clinical research trials on prayer reflect good-hearted attempts to drag spirituality into the research sphere, but, so far, as explained in Chapter 5, they have been unconvincing and possibly ill conceived. They have failed to produce acceptable "evidence" and may be about to vanish. For doctors, miracles cannot happen; they ignore the saints, both in practical terms of the clinic and in the abstract of the laboratory. But given how people use them, the saints support medical science.

How can we account for this vast discrepancy between the people who pray and the physicians who ignore? Are most doctors not paying attention to what goes on in the lives and minds of their patients? Are they consumed with the power of their objective observation or subjective impressions of the sick? Are patients not telling their doctors how they experience their suffering and their struggle to recover?

Why Do Physicians Ignore Miracles and Prayer?

First, doctors are uncomfortable with death. Equating the utility of all spiritual appeals for healing with successful outcomes—the miracle—reduces the power of faith and the role of saints to a tiny tip of an iceberg—insignificant and dismissible. Most such appeals do not result in cures, although they still serve a purpose. By the time I had finished the book on miracles, I saw that death was a major player in the workings of both medicine and religion. These parallel human endeavors rely on highly evolved bodies of wisdom to read signs in individuals confronted with the same problems. Medicine is to alleviate suffering and postpone death; religion is to console us to their inevitability. The ritualistic similarities described in the last chapter show that they have parallels in practice as well as intent.

But medicine can never fully achieve its goals, because at some point it will fail—for everyone. We all must die. In the main, pilgrims pray hoping for a miracle, but they are also preparing for the end. Notwithstanding the advent of specialists in ethics and palliative care, physicians deal poorly with death because it is the enemy that pervades medical endeavor. This discomfort may even explain the relatively recent creation of clinical specialties for "end-of-life issues" in order to allow the rest of us to ignore this unpleasant matter. Priests are more comfortable; for them death is a form of rebirth, possibly even an opportunity. Sometimes, patients too are more realistic about their poor prognoses than their doctors seem to appreciate.

As the MEDLINE survey showed, a few medical professionals actually want to deflect patients from expecting or craving the supernatural so that they will receive proper care and not abuse resources. However, were those doctors to listen to the stories labeled "miracles," either from the surveys or the Vatican archives, they would find that their worries of unrealistic expectations or neglect of orthodox treatments are unfounded. The miracles identified by pilgrims have little to do with the supernatural or the breaking of natural laws; they involve reassurance, encouragement, assistance, and healing in the context of orthodox medical and surgical care. Some involve advising patients to simply accept the doctors' advice. After all, for the devout, medicine is just another divine gift (Figure 1.3). God helps those who help themselves (and others). And most people who pray do not expect healing at all; they seek comfort, consolation, courage, and strength. While nearly half of the pilgrims surveyed had heard of miracles, most had not experienced one themselves; yet they continue to pray and believe. Skeptical physicians might be surprised to learn that the saints are on their side (Figure 6.1).

Second, in fairness, we do not want or expect doctors to recommend prayer; we want them to understand and believe in earthly cures. Patients have always known that the doctor would prescribe material remedies rather than pilgrimage and prayer. Since the time of Hippocrates in the fifth century BC, western medicine has self-consciously defined itself by its opposition to supernatural causes and cures. In the treatise "The Sacred Disease," the Hippocratic author wrote about the condition now known as epilepsy: "It is not in my opinion, any more divine or sacred than other diseases, but has a natural cause, and its supposed divine origin is due to men's inexperience and their wonder at its peculiar character."[3] The early church has been described as a healing religion opposed to medicine. Why? Because the church was opposed to magic, and medicine was a pagan profession, therefore magical; however, other scholars suggest that this apparent hostility has been overblown.[4] Clearly some kind of tension lurked in the background. Legend holds that one of the early doctor saints, Orestes, was charged with practicing magic, as if it was a crime; another, Cyprian, is said to have been a pagan magician before he took up Christianity and medicine, as if repudiating one was tantamount to repudiating the other. It is striking how many of those early doctor saints were "unmercenary" (Anargyroi), like Cosmas and Damian (Table 8).

In Christian-dominated Europe, wise doctors made room for God, but they occupied entirely different spheres.[5] The sixteenth-century surgeon

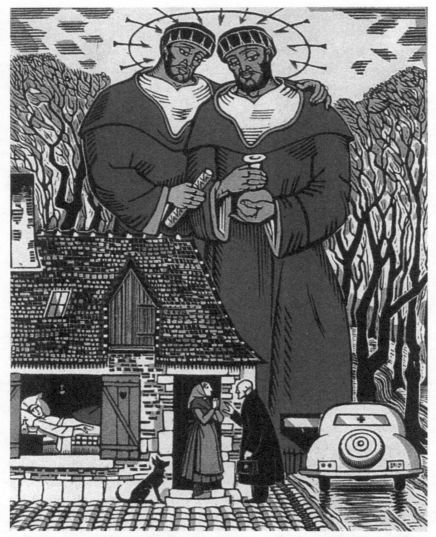

FIGURE 6.1 Visit to the patient. Jean Chièze, 1942. Collection Pierre Julien—William Helfand.

Ambroise Paré wrote, "I bandage them, but God heals them." Two centuries later, Benjamin Franklin added cynicism to the dyad: "God heals, and the Doctor takes the Fees."[6] The Enlightenment intelligentsia ascribed belief in miracles to popular traditions of the uneducated, while Protestants argued that miracles had ceased with the New Testament.[7] A medical student in late nineteenth-century Belgium stated the skeptical position so well that he was cited by a Canadian medical journal in 1880: "To believe in miracles one would have to be drunk."[8] Physicians tried to respect religion, but they did not practice it in the clinical realm.

In the mid-twentieth century, the gap between science and religion grew even wider. Science had become god-like, and the public generally shared physicians' confidence in its promise. But now, in this so-called *post*modern world, society has grown skeptical of science and statistics, while medicine remains relentlessly positivistic, confident in its numbers and commitment to the material world, even when it attempts to address the spiritual. For scientists, then, the miraculous cannot exist because supernatural events necessarily transgress the laws of nature—laws that cannot be broken, according to the scientific paradigm. Divine intervention is against medical teaching, and it is also against how society expects doctors to behave. My early assimilation of this message as a student explains the lingering sense of discomfort so long ago after I told a religious woman that she might pray to Saint Marguerite d'Youville.

Third, physicians confronted with claims of divine intervention tend to equate miracles with magic. For some, a miracle "must be" understood as a manifestation of God or the supernatural.[9] This view poses an enormous problem for atheist practitioners invited to think about unexplained things of wonder; however, for others, God may not be essential to a definition of miracle that relies on the occurrence of scientifically inexplicable events. For one scholar at least, miracles might actually be evidence against the existence of God.[10] Intrigued by the mutability of science itself, another suggested that "claims to the *scientific* impossibility" of miracles were "outmoded" and that they emerged from "complete intellectual vacuousness . . . no matter how distinguished the authority."[11] It boils down to a clash between world views and interpretation. With no dispute over what took place, agreement can never be reached between the religious and the nonreligious on how to interpret it.[12]

When I first began this work, I discovered that magic is often discussed in a context of miracles. Intriguingly, even useful distinctions can be made between miracles and magic; however, I eventually decided that the concept of magic was not helpful because none of those involved in either medicine or religion would embrace it as their own.[13] Nevertheless, suspicions of magic pervade medical views of reported miracles, dragging a host of undeserved negative connotations with it: illusion, deception, sensationalism, and fraud. It may even invoke a kind of professional duplicity, as if a patient committed to spiritual healing cannot also be devoted to her doctor. Doctors reject magic, and if they think miracles have something to do with it, they reject miracles too.

In the end, after all this work, I realized that praying to Cosmas and Damian may well be about health and medicine, but it is not for the purpose of miracles and healing. The medical saints are Brother Mark's companions on the final journey that we all must take. Cosmas and Damian are relevant not only for bridging a gap with their doctoring in the context of faith and mortality, but also, and perhaps more importantly, because of their death.

Why Are Miracles Mostly about Illness?

Why do pilgrims rarely report other types of miracles, such as conversions, provision of food, walking on water, or visions? On some level, this is a theological question. If people are true believers, shouldn't they accept God's will, allow disease to take its course, embrace their sufferings, and face the end with equanimity? Why should they be so egotistical as to imagine that God or a saint would take a personal interest in their plight? Isn't it contradictory or hypocritical to try to delay one's entry into heaven? I have no definite answer to these questions. To a physician, however, it seems natural enough to want to stay alive for as long as possible. Here are some of my thoughts as to why transcendence appears in the setting of illness—not only for Cosmas and Damian, but for all the saints.

First, doctors are obliged to toe the line about the natural boundaries of science, but ordinary people are not constrained to follow any one practice; nor must they heed narrow definitions of transcendent experience. Sick people partake of all the traditions around them. Seeing a doctor has never precluded consulting a saint. Since the earliest times, societies have kept a place for parallel forms of religious healing. Even Hippocratic medicine was used by both Christians and pagans in a manner that complemented and interpreted the articles of their faith.[14] Ours does too. People may consult physicians and carefully follow their advice, but they simultaneously look for other ways out of their sickness. They may see their doctors as *instruments* of healing, but they are equally comfortable with, if not more inclined to, the opinion that cures are effected by a deity or a saint. And mostly they do not tell: filled with the age-old desire to please and be liked, patients protect the doctor by catering to her presumed need to believe in her craft; claiming that prayers "work" too just might offend.

Second, ordinary people today understand that medicine sometimes made dreadful mistakes, and mistakes could happen again. They are suspicious of arrogance and exclusivity in health-care providers. The medical hegemony of the mid-twentieth century turns out to have been a short-lived blip, deviating from a long tradition of health-care pluralism that is now being revived. Given the first proposition above about doctors' confidence in their craft, the *fallibility* of medicine, only grudgingly acknowledged by its practitioners, also becomes a reason to pray.

Third, evidence-based statistics and RCTs about large cohorts mean little for individuals. People want personalized answers and they want limitless hope when nothing else is available. A solemn statement that offers fifty-fifty odds is not good enough. Evidence-Based Medicine's emphasis on numbers generated by large cohorts—together with its reticence to promise—provides yet another reason to pray.

Fourth, with respect to the miracles used in the canonization process, the involvement of doctors constitutes a kind of third-party witness unavailable to most other types of miracles. Those other moments of transcendence—visions, food, conversions—may well occur, but they will have no witnesses at all. The physician's detachment and supposed objectivity—or even better, her religious skepticism—offer a touchstone for authorities seeking to avoid being duped by enthusiasms of the faithful. Remarkably, then, medical skepticism keeps the church focused on physical healing in its quest for evidence of the divine.

Fifth and last, spiritual healing reclaims patient ownership over experience. The disease concepts that doctors use in diagnosis and treatment are defined and detected by complex—dare I say miraculous?—technologies aimed at the least, material change. The patient's story has become far less important; sometimes it is not needed at all. This narrow concept of disease excludes the sick, stripping them of control when they want to participate in their own attempts at recovery. This problem is at the root of recent attempts to revive "patient-centeredness" in medical teaching and care. In contrast, a miracle story places the patient at the center of her diagnosis and treatment; it assigns agency. In a sense, a miracle story is also the construction of a disease concept; and therapies must be consistent with perceived causes and symptoms. A cure will not "work" unless it addresses these personal notions too.[15] If a person believes that her illness is a product of unexpiated sin, she will not be cured without the "right" treatment, which may entail sacrifice, pilgrimage, and prayer, as well as chemotherapy. Getting better is directly connected to personal gestures of supplication, penance, thanksgiving, and worship. Denying the integral importance of these ideas in a patient's experience perpetuates that gulf between the reductionism of medicine and the holism of life. It is these personal gestures of appeal to medicine and beyond that provide a link to the illness and healing experience of all people, whether they are religious or not.

Cosmas and Damian of Toronto

Finally we can answer that question: what are Cosmas and Damian doing in Toronto? They are Roman Catholic saints popular with people of southern Italian origin who live in the parish of Saint Francis of Assisi Church. The veneration in Utica by the descendants of immigrants from Alberobello served as a reminder and a stimulus. The statues were brought in 1987 by a devoted parishioner who had emigrated from near Isernia, where veneration of the santi medici dates back to the twelfth century or earlier; she had also attended the Utica feast. The saints and their statues fit perfectly with the trappings of Italian feste in general—celebration, faith, hope, and inspiration to acts of charity. Locally, their presence conformed to the range of prior performative events within the yearly cycle of that parish. They provide a pretext for social cohesion, preserve tradition, invite worship and thanksgiving, and symbolize family and selfless service. This study has demonstrated support for the theories of diffusion, genealogy, and sociology.

But there are some interesting challenges in the observations. The feast emerged later than the first waves of immigration, suggesting that forces beyond nostalgia and direct diffusion were at play. Not all the pilgrims who celebrate the saints are from Italy. Indeed, at each site some visitors were neither Italian nor Catholic, and their ancestors may never have heard of the saints. Also challenging the genealogical theory was the presence of Haitian immigrants at Italian feasts, people whose genuine devotion to Cosmas and Damian may have harkened back to forgotten African beliefs or been sparked more recently by their cultural penchant to pilgrimage. The presence of divine twins in these communities and in other traditions, such as Japanese and Amerindian mythology, suggests that the santi medici may represent recurring dichotomies that are universally noticed and respected within the human mind. This observation lends support to the psychoanalytic interpretations of why the twin deities are celebrated as healers now and at other times and places.

The trappings of the feste followed small variations on the main theme of masses, processions, prayer, and fun, but the devotion was not restricted to those activities, nor even to that time of year. Some were more "medical" than others or than their parent events in Italy. Fully exploding my notion that the

value-added medicalization of Cosmas and Damian was a New World attribute, the activities in Bitonto and Rome bespeak a special concern in the
Old World to demonstrate the relevance of the santi medici to modern medicine and society on a global scale. The veneration is not static.

And the saints are at work. Cosmas and Damian turn out to be active
consultants in a health-care smorgasbord. The separation of medicine and
religion is an artifact of scholarship. For the Ersilia Jannettas and Joe DeCan-
dias of this world, they are one. And they are one for thousands who find help
from these and other saints at healing shrines around the world. Perhaps medicine and faith are united not only for this particular social group, but also for
those who eat tofu, run marathons, practice yoga, watch their weight, curb
their diets, play sports, and take multivitamins or antioxidants. These people
are pilgrims too—hedging their bets against the inevitable.

So—with its failings, skepticism, and statistics, medicine creates space,
even a need, for the saints. To counter its indifferent probabilities and cold
technology, the saints promise hope against hope. Ironically, then, it may be
the miracle of scientific medicine that provides greatest impetus for the continuing miracles of faith. Herein may lie the best explanation for how, on a
specific day next September, in the shadow of a university hospital, you will
find new statues of ancient twins making their way down a Toronto street.

Epilogue

I WROTE THE conclusion to this book in the summer of 2010. But by the next October, Canada was celebrating saints once again. Marguerite d'Youville's old rival, Brother André Bessette, was to be canonized as the second Canadian-born saint, along with Australia's first saint, Mary MacKillop. The miracle that had been used in his cause was finally revealed. Unsurprisingly, it was another spectacular healing from physical illness. In 1999 a nine-year-old boy was struck by a car while riding his bicycle and sustained a terrible head injury. He lay in a deep coma. Doctors did not expect him to live, at least not without severe problems. But prayers asking Brother André to intercede on the lad's behalf were soon followed by his complete recovery. Now a young man of nineteen, he did not want attention or publicity, and the grateful family tasked Father Grou of St. Joseph's Oratory in Montreal to be their spokesman. Even without more details, I knew that the lad's doctors had cooperated with the investigation and that the Vatican experts had been satisfied that his recovery was scientifically inexplicable.

Hundreds of Canadians (and Australians) booked tickets for Rome. Reporters unfamiliar with the process scrambled to find "talking heads" to fill air space and help interpret this extraordinary manifestation of faith, inspired by an unpretentious and probably illiterate brother who had been dead for seventy-three years. Always trolling for attention, my university beamed me out as an "expert on miracles," based on the 2009 book. For a brief moment, I was suddenly in demand for national and local channels of radio and television as well as documentary film companies in both official languages. Most interviewers simply wanted to know how the canonization process worked; many were surprised that it could still be going after all these centuries; some doubted my word that medical science could be seriously involved.

At least two famous and normally well-respected pundits (who clearly had not read my book) grew impatient with the fuss and pronounced the whole business a bunch of foolishness. "Amused" by the media hype devoted to "this type of superstitious guff," one wrote that "people would be a lot better off if they put their faith in science rather than holy oil."[1] The other seemed bent on stomping out religion altogether; he belittled the Vatican's attempts to verify miracles as an appeal to "pseudo-scientific twaddle."[2] Ahem. That was me he was talking about, although he didn't know it.

Somehow, word got out that I was an atheist—"an atheist who believes in miracles." For a few interviewers, that sidebar became the main story, as if one belief was mutually incompatible with the other. Thus a talk-show host caught David and me in our car on the highway; we pulled over.

HE: Now doctor, I hear that you are an atheist, is that right?

ME: Yes.

HE: So, how can you believe in miracles if you don't believe in God?

ME: I think unexpected things can happen for which we have no scientific explanation. If someone else attributes it to God, I have no problem with that.

HE: But how do *you* explain it?

ME: I can't, that's the whole point.

HE: But how do you *explain* it?

ME: I can't.

We grew equally exasperated with each other on live radio while baffled, homeward-bound drivers switched channels.

Once again, I realized that the word "miracle" somehow has come to belong exclusively to God. Yet what a shame that we "scientists" (and "twaddlers") do not allow ourselves to indulge in wonder too. When confronted with the amazing and the inexplicable, why can't we allow people to tell their own stories?

Historians of medicine are used to quietude; even our most controversial work is usually ignored. But by the end of that weekend, I had made fourteen appearances at odd hours of day and night, from the campus radio or television stations. It was daunting, especially since slippage from the main topic was an occupational hazard: no predicting when I'd suddenly be asked to justify the barbarity of the Crusaders or the shameful deeds of abusing priests. The last television interview happened late on the night of the canonization; it was dark and cold, and dry leaves were swirling round the empty parking lot. Shivering and relieved, I climbed in my car and switched on the engine, as the radio sprang to life at CBC where it always sits—and an odiously familiar voice was going on about miracles and science. They were replaying a morning show.

In contrast to the ignoring of doctors and scientists and the scorn of militant, atheist scribblers, the public clearly cares about this topic. One of the best things about all the attention was a warm e-mail greeting from Lise Normand, alive and well, and the only person I have ever met who could write, "I did have leukemia more than 30 years ago." Her miracle. Mine too.

I still keep one of Jeanne's 8 x 10 glossies of Jean Paul II and me framed on my office wall. Students eye it carefully, but only a few muster the courage to ask about it. When they do, the conversation usually runs something like this:

STUDENT: I'm a little surprised to see that someone like you would be a devout Catholic.

ME: What do you mean "like you"?

STUDENT: Well, medicine and its history seem to make you skeptical.

ME: I'm not a Catholic, but I did meet the Pope once. Maybe history of medicine reminds us to be skeptical *and* open-minded.

STUDENT: I guess history has taken you to some interesting places.

ME: Yes, it has. But I didn't meet the Pope because of history. I met him because of hematology.

STUDENT: Oh, how is that?

ME: How long have you got?

Tables

Table 1 Founding and Responses to the Question: What are your origins?
How far have you come today?

	Toronto	Utica	Manhattan	Howard Beach	Cambridge	Total
Year						
Founded	1987	1912	1903	1977	1926	
Number	68	88	26	11	45	238
Female (%)	75	67		100	64.4	70.8[*]
Italian origin (%)	90	80	81	73	82	82.8
home (%)	70.5	45.5		100	62.2	
1 hr	19	19	96		20	
2 hr		2.3	4			
3 hr						
4 hr		1.2			13.3	
5 hr		28.4				
6 hr		2.3				
Further					4.4	

[*]Question overlooked in Manhattan; percent calculated here with total of 212

Table 2 Responses to the Questions: Is it important to you that the saints are twins? Doctors?

	Toronto	Utica	Manhattan	Howard Beach	Cambridge	Total
Number	68	88	26	11	45	238
Is important to you that the saints are						
Twins (%)	68.7	46.8	42.3	9	37.8	46
Doctors (%)	79	72.6	58.3	36.5	75.6	72

Table 3 Responses to the Question: Why do you attend the feast?

	Toronto	Utica	Manhattan	Howard Beach	Cambridge	Total
Number	68	88	26	11	45	238
Reasons (%)						
Fondness	47	59.1	34.6	63.6	60	53.1
Tradition	23.5	64.8	84.6	45.5	80	56.5
Friends	4.4	33	11.5	45.5	22.2	20.9
Parish	30	20.5	3.8	36.4	0	20.5
Other	16.2	6.8			15.2	10
Faith	1.5	1.1			2.2	1.3
Hope	1.5					0.4
Feast/fun	5.9	1.1	3.8		2.2	1.7
Healing		3.4				1.3
Shared name			3.7			0.8
Organizer/ band				9	4.4	1.3
History/ culture					8.9	1.7

Table 4 Responses to the Question: Have you attended other feast-day celebrations? Where?

	Toronto	Utica	Manhattan	Howard Beach	Cambridge	Total
Number	68	88	26	11	45	238
No (%)	36.7	56.8	19.2	81.8	37.8	44.5
Yes (%)	63.2	43.2	80.8	18.2	64.4	55.9
Where* (%)						
Italy	29.4	20.5	57.7	18.2	24.4	27.7
Toronto		9	3.8			3.8
Utica	26.5				15.6	10.5
Manhattan		2.3			8.9	2.5
H. Beach			11.5		2.2	1.7
Cambridge	1.5					0.4
Other or unspec.						
N. America	16.2	13.6	23.1		26.7	17.2

*Responses by place may total more than the percentages responding "yes" because many people had visited more than one site.

Table 5 Responses to the Question: Do you know of any miracles?

	Toronto	Utica	Manhattan	Howard Beach	Cambridge	Total
Number	68	88	26	11	45	238
Do you know of miracles (%)	46.8	46.6	42.3	18.3	57.8	45.7

Table 6 Summary of Miracles following appeals to SS Cosmas and Damian as told by pilgrims

Source	Subject	Miracle
		Toronto
Man age 35 (a twin)	mother	hospital, medal "helped possibly physically and definitely spiritually"
Man age 50	priest	Cancer, healing of
Woman age 50	self	cancer given 3 months; but cured

(*continued*)

Table 6 (*continued*)

Source	Subject	Miracle
Woman age 50	brother	heart disease had surgery; mother prayed for him
Woman age 70	sister-in-law's mother	in hospital awaiting surgery in Isernia; vision of saints operating on her; surgery not needed; died age 89
Woman age 70	self	saints granted wish for her health
Woman age 70	son	arm paralyzed from birth; used wax votive; cured
Woman age 40	self	heart condition; afraid of tonsillectomy; saints reassured her; cured with operation
Woman age 50	mother	in hospital in Italy awaiting operation; saints reassured her; cured with surgery; lived 10 years.
Woman, age 60	husband	heart disease; prayed for him at Utica
Woman age 30	friend's mother	healing

Manhattan

Source	Subject	Miracle
Man	wife	recovery from operation for cancer
Woman, elderly	grandmother	breast cancer in hospital; saints in dream cured before surgery, lived to age 90
Woman	mother	breast cancer surgery
	uncle	3 operations on spine and stomach
	uncle	cardiac surgery; lived 40 more years
Man, elderly	sister	pain and weight loss; exploratory surgery
woman, elderly	friend's son	dying of fever; his mother prayed; even doctors say recovery is a miracle and they contribute to the feast day every year

Utica

Source	Subject	Miracle
Man b. 1922	self	diphtheria age 4
Woman age 65	self	open-heart surgery age 60; saints appeared in vision
Woman age 50	self	Carcinoid tumor cured
	woman	brain tumor; surgery found no lesion
	friend's grandson	blindness

Table 6   (*continued*)

Source	Subject	Miracle
Woman	father	car accident; unharmed; saints image on windshield
Woman	friend	inability to walk, cured.
Woman	son	Ewing's sarcoma; resolved after prayer
Man age 50	self	healed from illness after priest prayed
Woman age 30	uncle Nick	Rheumatic fever as child; father hitchhiked to feast
	male cousin	football head injury; his grandmother bought statues; put on his bed
Man age 50	self (Nick's son)	head injury age 17; still has statues; attends feast (same miracle as above)
Woman age 70	mother	coma for two weeks; family appealed; lived 17 years

Howard Beach

Source	Subject	Miracle
Woman	woman in Italy	healed of illness by devotion
Mother	twin sons	serious illness; treated by doctors in hospital; attends feast annually

Cambridge, Mass.

Source	Subject	Miracle
Woman age 57	man, a builder	urinary problem; told to pray by 2 strangers; attends feast annually
	fisherman in Gaeta	learned he had cancer; met 2 men on beach who told him to pray; cured. Others knew same story
Woman age 60	self	complicated labor; Cesarean; vision
	self	kidney failure, needing dialysis; cured
Woman	father	cardiac arrest; lived 2 more years
	husband	pulmonary emboli; recovered
	mother	massive stroke; image of saints comforted at time of her death
Man age 55	wife	cancer of uterus given 6 months; radiation and to chemotherapy 10 years ago; still alive
Woman age 60	husband	bleeding ulcer, 50/50 chance; 2 surgeries
Woman age 70	male cousin	dying of typhoid; family prayed; gold votives
	self	ill in bed; vision of saints; attends annually

(*continued*)

Table 6 (*continued*)

Source	Subject	Miracle
Woman age 60	father age 51	appendicitis, peritonitis; dream of saints; surgery; still alive late 70s
Man b. 1928	self	pneumonia age 9 months; mother and aunt prayed
Man age 35	great-grandfather	blindness owing to eye injury; attends feast
Woman age 50	daughter	ankle fracture; operation pinned "for life"; prayed; pins removed; healed
Woman age 35	self	mammogram breast lump; prayed; lump vanished
Woman age 77	brother	boat accident; fractured arm during war
	self	crushed arm; pins; doctors operated
	male friend	cancer, dying; dream of saints; healed

Table 7 Towns with shrines dedicated to the medical saints in Puglia*

Bari
To west
   Bartletta
   Trani
   Canosa
   Ruvo
   Terlizzi
   Molfetta
   Bitonto
   Toritto
   Altamura
To the east
   Turi
   Conversano
   Putignano
   Alberobello
   Noci
   Fasano
   Locorotondo
   Monopoli
   Ostuni
   Brindisi

Table 7 (*continued*)

Taranto and vicinity
    Massafra
    Ginosa
    Laterza
    S. Marzano di S. Gioseppe
    Monteparano
    Fragagnano
    Torricella
    Mandu
    Bisceglieria
    Guangano

Lecce and south
    Nardò
    Gallipoli
    Sannicola
    Alezio
    Taviano
    Ugento
    Corsano
    Diso
    Poggiardo
    Uggiano la Chiesa
    Muro Leccese
    Maglie
    Cannole

*special thanks to Pierre Julien

Table 8 Doctor saints

A. Pre-Congregation Physicians, Healers, and Hospital Founders

Aemilianus the martyr, 5th C

Agapitus of Kiev, 11th C

Alexander of Phrygia, martyr of Lyon, 2nd C

Alquirino Cistercian monk, 12th C

Antiochus of Mauritania, 2nd C

Antiochus of Sebaste, Armenia, early 4th C

Asia (Mar Ishaa of Antioch), 4th C

Bartholomew the Apostle, 1st C

Basil of Caesarea, 4th C

Benedict Crispus of Milan, 8th C

Bernardino of Siena, d. 1444

Blaise of Sebaste, Armenia, 4th C

Caesarius of Nazianzen, 4th C

Carponius (Calpurnio) of Rome, 3rd C

Cassian of Todi, 4th C

Codratus of Corinth, 3rd C

Cyprian of Antioch, late 3rd C

Cyrus of Alexandria, 4th C

Diomedes of Tarsus, 3rd C

Dionisio diacono, 5th C

Dionysius of Rome, 3rd C

Elizabeth of Hungary, 13th C

Eusebius, Pope, 4th C

Fulbert of Chartes, 11th C

Gennadius of Constantinople, 5th C

Hermolaus of Nicodemia, 3rd C

Hildegard of Bingen, 12th C

Ivo of Chartres, 12th C

John Damascene, 8th C

Julian (Elian) of Emesa, Syria, 4th C

Julian of Cyprus, 3rd C

Juvenal of Narni, 4th C

Lanfranco of Pavia and Canterbury, 11th C

Leonilla of Cappadocia, 2nd C

Table 8 (*continued*)

Leontius & Carpophoros of Vicenza, 4th C
Liberatus of Carthage, 5th C
Luke the Evangelist, 1st C
Lutgarde of Aywieres, 13th C
Medico of Otrocoli, 2nd C
Nicarete (Niceras) of Constantinople, 5th C
Orestes of Cappadocia, 3rd C
Pantaleon of Nicomedia, 3rd C
Papilus of Pergamon, 3rd C
Paul of Merida, 6th C
Paul the Greek, physician, 3rd C
Ravenne and Rasiphe of Bayeux, 4th C
Saint Sanctus of Lyons, 2nd C
Sampson the Hospitable, 6th C
Thallelaius (Talaleo) of Aegea, 3rd C
Theodosia of Caesarea, 4th C
Theodotus of Laodicea, Syria, 4th C
Ursicinus of Ravenna, 3rd C
Victor III (Desiderius), 11th C
Vilfère (Vulferius, Gouffier) of Auxerre, 9th C
William Firmatus of Tours, 12th C
Zenaide and Philonille of Tarsus, 1st C
Zenobius of Aegea, 3rd C
Zenobius of Sidon, 4th C

B. Post-Congregation Medical Saints

	Born	Died	Canonized or Beatified
Saints			
Antonio Maria Zaccaria	1502	1539	1897
Filippo Benizi	1233	1285	1671
Francesca Romana	1384	1440	1608
Francis of Nagasaki		1597	1862
Giana Beretta Molla	1922	1962	2004
Giuseppe Moscati	1880	1927	1987
Joachim Sakakibara of Japan		1613	1862
Joseph Canh of Vietnam	1763	1838	1988
Martin Porres	1579	1639	1962

(*continued*)

Table 8 (*continued*)

René Goupil	1608	1642	1930
Riccardo Pampuri	1837	1930	1989
Blesseds			
Antonio della Torre of Milan	1424	1494	1897
Bertharius of Monte Cassino, 9th C			1727
Gabriel of St. Magdalen		1632	1892
Giles of Santarem, Portugal	1185	1265	1748
John Juvenal Ancina	1545	1603	1890
Mark of Montegallo	1426	1497	1839
Niels Stensen	1638	1686	1988

Notes

CHAPTER 1

1. Lambertini, *De servorum Dei*, 1734–38; Duffin, *Medical Miracles*, 2009, 11–35; Higgins, *Stalking the Holy*, 2006, 27-78; Woodward, *Making Saints*, 1990, 73–86.
2. Evensen and Stavem, "Long-Term Survival," 1986; Gale and Foon, "Acute Myeloid Leukemia," 1986; Keating et al., "Improved Prospects," 1982; Schwartz et al., "Multivariate Analysis," 1984; Whittaker et al., "Long-Term Survival," 1981.
3. Ferland-Angers, *Mère d'Youville*, 1945.
4. Ferland-Angers, *Mère d'Youville*, 1945, 38.
5. Congregatio pro causis sanctorum, *Marianopolitana*, 1989.
6. Anon., "Grey Nuns Founder," 1990.

CHAPTER 2

1. My translation from "L'affluence des malades au Cosmidion n'a pas résulté de quelque souvenir du paganisme, mais d'un mouvement essentiel de l'âme humaine; en tout temps, et quelles que fussent les croyances, ce mouvement devait conduire aux Guérisseurs, quelque nom qu'ils aient porté. . . . et tous les guérisseurs possibles ont repondu a ces deux faits constants, la misère humaine, la confiance incoercible dans les celestes Evergètes."
2. Bagnell, *Canadese*, 1989; Eisenbichler, *Italian Region*, 1998; Harney, "Toronto's Little Italy," 1981; Iacovetta, *Such Hard-Working People*, 1992; Jansen, *Factbook*, 1987; Jansen, *Italians*, 1988; Stanger-Ross, *Staying Italian*, 2009; Zucchi, *Italians in Toronto*, 1988.
3. Deubner, *Kosmas und Damian*, [1907] 1980, esp. epigraph citing Le Nain de Tillemont. See also Baring-Gould, "Cosmas and Damian," 1914; David-Danel, *Iconographie*, 1958; Delehaye, "Recueil antique," 1925, 8–18; Delehaye, *Legends*, 1962; Festugière, *Sainte Thècle, Saints Côme et Damien*, 1971, 98–213; Julien and Ledermann, *Saint Côme et Saint Damien*, 1985; Julien et al., *Cosma e Damiano*,

1993; Skrobucha, *Patrons*, 1965; Stiltingo, "SS Cosma, Damiano," *Acta Sanctorum*, 1760; Thurston, and Attwater, "Cosmas and Damian," 1963; Wittmann, *Kosmas und Damian*, 1967.

4. Voragine, "Cosmas and Damian,"1969; Stiltingo, "SS Cosma, Damiano," *Acta Sanctorum*, 1760, 474–475; Festugière, *Sainte Thècle, Saints Côme et Damian*, 1971, 100, 149.

5. Ball, *Rome in the East*, 2000, 163–164; Frézouls, "Recherches," 1954–55; Shahid, "Arab-Christian Pilgrimages," 1998; Sournia and Sournia, *L'orient des premiers chrétiens*, 1966.

6. Brown, *Cult of the Saints*, 1981, 7; Risse, *Mending Bodies*, 1999, 79; Temkin, *Hippocrates*, 1991, 75, 80.

7. Theodoret, *Thérapeutique*, 1958. See also Adnès and Canivet, "Guérisons," 1967; Borella, *Le mystère*, 1989, 38–39; Temkin, *Hippocrates*, 1991, 145.

8. Deubner, *Kosmas und Damian*, [1907] 1980, 81.

9. Hamilton, *Incubation*, 1906, esp. 119–127; Csepregi, "Mysteries," 2005; Delehaye, *Legends*, 1962, 121–122; Jackson, *Doctors and Diseases*, 1988, 145–159; Risse, *Mending Bodies*, 57–58; Rousselle, "Healing Cults," 1985; Sudhoff, "Healing Miracles," 1926; Temkin, *Hippocrates*, 1991, 76, 80, 183–184.

10. Kazhdan, *Oxford Dictionary*, 1991, vol. 2, 1083; Malamut, *Sur la route*, 1993, 527–565; Procopius, *Buildings* (VI, 5–8), vol. 7, 62–63; Krueger, "Christian Piety," 2005; Horden, "Saints and Doctors," 1982; Marraffa, *Santi Cosma e Damiano*, 2000, 133; Miller, *Birth of the Hospital*, 1985, 124.

11. Deubner, *Kosmas und Damian*, [1907] 1980; Festugière, *Sainte Thècle, Saints Côme et Damian*, 1971, 98–213; Rupprecht, *Cosmae et Damiani*, 1935. See also Csepregi, "Mysteries," 2005.

12. Delehaye, *Legends*, 1962, 122; Festugière, *Sainte Thècle, Saints Côme et Damian*, 1971, 88–89.

13. Deubner, *Kosmas und Damian*, [1907] 1980, 164–166, 201–202 ("wunders" 25, 43); Festugière, *Sainte Thècle, Saints Côme et Damian*, 1971, 91, 98–213, esp. 160–161, 203, (miracles 25, 43); Stiltingo, "SS Cosma, Damiano," *Acta Sanctorum*, 1760, 467 (miracle 25).

14. Zimmerman collected forty different images of the black leg miracle, from the fourteenth century to the twentieth. *One Leg in the Grave*, 1998. See also Barkan, "Cosmas and Damian," 1996; Huisman, "Human Frailty," 1998; Stiltingo, "SS Cosma, Damiano," *Acta Sanctorum*, 1760, 461.

15. Kahan, "Cosmas and Damian," 1983; Lehrman, "Miracle," 1994.

16. Schlich, "How Gods and Saints Became Transplant Surgeons," 1995, 311.

17. Risse, *Mending Bodies*, 79–83.

18. Kazhdan, *Oxford Dictionary*, 1991, vol. 2, 1083.

19. Festugière, *Vie de Theodore*, 1970, vol. 2, 37–38; Malamut, *Sur la route*, 1993, 212–215.

20. Labriola, *I santi Cosma e Damiano*, 1984, 34.

21. Tucci, "Eight Fragments," 2004.

22. Amundsen, "Medieval Christian Tradition," 1986, 79–80; Amundsen, *Medicine, Society, and Faith*, 1996, 176–178; Angenendt, *Heilige und Reliquien*, 1994, 149; Brown, *Cult of the Saints*, 1981, 88–94; Ferngren, *Medicine and Health Care*, 2009, 82–83.

23. Stiltingo, "SS Cosma, Damiano," *Acta Sanctorum*, 1760, 442–443.

24. Adam of Bremen, *History*, 1959, 61; Stiltingo, "SS Cosma, Damiano," *Acta Sanctorum*, 1760, 447–448, 452.

25. David-Danel, "Les lieux de culte," 1966, 215–216; David-Danel, *Répertoire*, [ca 1969]; Stiltingo, "SS Cosma, Damiano," *Acta Sanctorum*, 1760, 446–447.

26. Matthews, "SS Cosmas and Damian," 1968.

27. Stiltingo, "SS Cosma, Damiano," *Acta Sanctorum*, 1760, 441–453, 458–459, esp. 459; Baring-Gould, "Cosmas and Damian," 1914, 400–401; Wittmann, *Kosmas und Damian*, 80–81.

28. David-Danel, *Iconographie*, 1958, 215–225; David-Danel, "Les lieux de culte," 1966; David-Danel, *Répertoire*, [ca 1969].

29. Wittmann, *Kosmas und Damian*, 82–118.

30. Labriola, *I santi Cosma e Damiano*, 1984, 38. My translation.

31. Labriola, *I santi Cosma e Damiano*, 1984, 22–23.

32. Lowe, *Nuns' Chronicles*, 2003, 61–71, 370–371.

33. Caraffa, *San Cosimato*, 1971; Lloyd and Einaudi, *SS. Cosma e Damiano in Mica Aurea*, 1998.

34. Vilarrasa i Coch, *Els Sants Metges*, 2004, 56–59.

35. Julien et al., *Cosma e Damiano*, 1993, lists on endpapers. Another list appeared at the website, Santi Cosma e Damiano, Basilica Santi Medici, Alberobello, http://www.basilicalberobello.com/?page_id=14, accessed June 30, 2010.

36. Thurston and Attwater, "Cosmas and Damian," 1963, 660.

37. Temperini, *Basilica*, nd, 33; Tucci, "Revival," 2004.

38. David-Danel, *Iconographie*, 1958, 107–123, esp. 113; Julien, "La confrérie," 1973; Julien, *Saint Côme et Saint Damian, patrons*, 1980; Pecker, ed. *La médecine à Paris*, 1984, 18–22, 105.

39. David-Danel, "Saint Côme," 1985.

40. David-Danel, *Iconographie*, 1958, 191–206, esp. 206.

41. Giannarelli, *Cosma e Damiano*, 2002.

42. Holmes, *Fra Filippo Lippi*, 1999, 125, 192–196.

43. See for example, Cannito, *I Santi Medici*, 1998; Marraffa, *Santi Cosma e Damiano*, 2000; Martellotta, *Memorie istoriche*, 1986; Pazzano and Capponi, *I Santi Medici*, 2000; Temperini, *Santi Cosma e Damiano*, 1997; Vacca, *Reading*, 1982; Zuring, *De heilige genezers*, 1989.

44. See for example, Deubner, *Kosmas und Damian*, [1907] 1980; Rupprecht, *Cosmae et Damiani*, 1935.

45. Wittmann, *Kosmas und Damian*, 1967, 32–37, 244.

46. Julien, "Côme et Damien," 1985, 50. My translation.

47. Brown, *Cult of the Saints*, 1981, 5–8; Cotter, *Miracles in Greco-Roman Antiquity*, 1999, 17–24, 54–73; Ferngren, *Medicine and Health Care*, 2009, 30–31, 41, 70–71; Hart, *Asclepius*, 2000, 183–186; Jones and Pennick, *History of Pagan Europe*, 1995, 104–105, 160–162, 193–194; Kee, *Medicine, Miracle, and Magic*, 1986, 118–120; Remus, *Pagan Christian Conflict*, 1983, 105–135; Temkin, *Hippocrates*, 1991, 75, 80, 167.

48. Albert, *Le culte de Castor et Pollux*, 1882; Harris, *The Dioscuri*, 1903; Ward, *Divine Twins*, 1968; Ward, "Separate Functions," 1970.

49. Father Gregory, Toronto, September 1996; Father F. J. Evans, Howard Beach, N.Y., August 12, 1998; Brother Mark McBride, Rome, June 19, 2010.

50. Dasen, *Jumeaux, jumelles*, 2005.

51. Cotter, *Miracles in Greco-Roman Antiquity*, 1999, 131, 134; Deubner, *Kosmas und Damian*, [1907] (1980), 113–117 ("wunder" 9); Festugière, *Sainte Thècle, Saints Côme et Damian*, 1971, 91, 110–112 (miracle 9).

52. Deubner, *Kosmas und Damian*, [1907] (1980), 201–203 ("wunders" 43, 44); Festugière, *Sainte Thècle, Saints Côme et Damian*, 1971, 204–205 (miracles 44, 45).

53. Brown, *Cult of the Saints*, 1981; Theodoret, *Thérapeutique*, 1958, 2: 335 (liber viii).

54. Festugière, *Sainte Thècle, Saints Côme et Damien*, 1971, 217–237; Montserrat, "Pilgrimage," 1998; Sudhoff, "Healing Miracles," 1926.

55. Harris, *Dioscuroi*, 1903, 62–63. On Chrysostom and medicine, see also, Amundsen, *Medicine, Society, and Faith*, 1996, 135; Ferngren, *Medicine and Health Care*, 2009, 78–79, 133; Risse, *Mending Bodies*, 1999, 73–87, 120–125, esp. 77–78; Temkin, *Hippocrates*, 1991, 139, 164, 220.

56. Ginzburg, *Cheese and the Worms*, 1980, 58.

57. Albert, *Le culte de Castor et Pollux*, 1882, esp. iv–v; Littleton, "Georges Dumézil," 1974; Littleton, *New Comparative Mythology*, 1982, 9–14; Schwartz, *Culture of the Copy*, 1996, 21–36; Ward, *Divine Twins*, 1968, 11, 15; Ward, "Separate Functions," 1970.

58. Krappe, *Mythologie universelle*, [1930] 1978, 63; Perrot, *Mythe et litterature*, 1976, 17.

59. Jones and Pennick, *History of Pagan Europe*, 1995, 118; Tacitus, *Germania*, 43; Ward, *Divine Twins*, 1968, 30–42.

60. Jones and Pennick, *History of Pagan Europe*, 1995, 144–146; Littleton, "Georges Dumézil," 1974; Littleton, *New Comparative Mythology*, 1982, 12; Ward, *Divine Twins*, 1968, 18, 28, 98n83.

61. Gärtner, *Theology of the Gospel of Thomas*, 1961, 96–97; Perrot, *Mythe et litterature*, 1976, 30; Pick, *Apocryphal Acts*, 1909, 226, 251–252.

62. Delehaye, "Castor et Pollux," 1904; Delehaye, *Legends of the Saints*, 1962, 125, 165n65.

63. Brown, *Cult of the Saints*, 1981, 5–6.

64. Festugière, *Sainte Thècle, Saints Côme et Damian*, 1971, 94–95. My translation.

65. On "degradation narrative," see Carroll, *American Catholics*, 2007, 93–95, 150–151.

66. Ferngren, "Early Christianity," 1992, 14; Ferngren, *Medicine and Health Care*, 2009, 45–48, esp. 85

67. Amundsen and Ferngren, "Early Christian Tradition," 1986, 55.

68. Carpenter, *Pagan and Christian Creeds*, 1971, 201–205; Festugière, *Sainte Thècle, Saints Côme et Damien*, 1971, 217–218.

69. Brown, *Cult of the Saints*, 1981, 18.

70. On these problems, see Van Dam, *Saints and their Miracles*, 1993, 84–86.

71. Stanger-Ross, *Staying Italian*, 2009, 76. See also Saint Francis of Assisi Church website http://www.stfrancis.ca/, accessed 29 October 2012.

72. Interview with Raffaele Paonessa, priest St. Lawrence the Martyr church, Scarborough, September 1991 and March 13, 1992.

73. Interview with Ersilia Jannetta and her daughter, Mary Colanardi, February 15, 1992.

74. Julien et al., *Cosma e Damiano*, 1993, 70–76.

75. Jansen, *Italians*, 1988, 57–75.

76. For summaries of these perspectives, see Larson, "Introduction," 1974; Littleton, "Georges Dumézil," 1974.

77. Krappe, *Mythologie universelle*, [1930] 1978, 53–100; Ward, *Divine Twins*, 1968, 3–7.

78. Hankoff, "Why the Healing Gods Are Twins," 1977.

79. Durkheim, "Definition of Religious Phenomena," [1899] 1975.

80. Gedda, *Twins*, 1961, 3–17; Schwartz, *Culture of the Copy*, 1996, 24; Tejirian, *Sexuality*, 1990, 208.

81. Gedda, *Twins*, 1961, 6–8; Judson, *Native Legends*, 2000, 40; Kroeber, *Native American Story Telling*, 2004, 62–63; Philippi, *Kojiki*, 1968, 48; Veith, "Twin Birth," 1960.

82. Jackson, *Doctors and Diseases*, 1988, 167–169; Travlos, *Pictorial Dictionary*, 1971, 127–137.

83. De Simoni, ed., *Ex voto*, 1986.

84. Grant, *Roman Forum*, 1970, 82–90.

85. Interview with Deacon William Dischiavo, July 18, 1994; Cimino, *St. Anthony of Padua Church*, 1987.

86. Vitucci Nicole, in mimeographed flyer and personal communication, Bill Dischiavo and Lorraine Bulson, secretary to the Congregation, Utica.

87. See for example, Simons, "Spiritual Values," 1993.

88. Iacovetta, *Such Hard-Working People*, 1992.

CHAPTER 3

1. Boobyer, "Gospel Miracles," 1964; Hardon, "Concept?" 1954; Université d'Angers, *Histoire des miracles*, 1983; Houston, *Reported Miracles*, 1994, 83–120; Larmer, *Water into Wine*, 1988, 93–109; Larmer, *Questions*, 1996; Perry, "Believing the Miracles," 1964; Peschel and Peschel, "Medical Miracles," 1988; Ramsey, "Miracles,"

[1952] 1964; Sabourin, *Divine Miracles*, 1977; Salleron, "Le miracle," 1983; Swinburne, *Concept*, 1970, 71.

2. O'Connell, "Roman Catholic Tradition," 1986.

3. Keller and Keller, *Miracles in Dispute*, 1969, 247.

4. Composta, *Il miracolo*, 1981; Darricau, "Une source," 1983; Viguerie, "Preface," 1983, 9–10; Viguerie, "Les caractères permanents," 1983; Resch, *Miracoli dei Beati, 1983–1990* and *1991–1995*, 2002; Resch, *Miracoli dei Santi*, 2002.

5. Cotter, *Miracles*, 1999, 175–178; Kee, *Medicine, Miracle, and Magic*, 1986, 3–4; Harrison, "Miracles, Early Modern Science," 2006; Lloyd, *Magic, Reason*, 1979; Mullin, *Miracles and Magic*, 1979, 66–83; Temkin, *Hippocrates*, 1991, 121–124, esp. 123; Thomas, *Religion*, 1971.

6. Temkin, *Hippocrates*, 1991, 121–124, esp. 123.

7. Durkheim, *Elementary Forms*, [1915] 1965, 57–63, 111.

8. Canguilhem, "Histoire des religions," 1964.

9. Eamon, "Technology as Magic," 1983; Green, "Surgeons and Shamans," 2006; Souverbie, "Magie et médecine," 1970; Webster, "Paracelsus," 1995.

10. Green, "Surgeons and Shamans," 2006; Hanson et al., "Providers," 2008; Preston, "Necessary Fictions," 1989; Risse, *Mending Bodies*, 1999, 683–684; Rossi et al., "Wizards," 1994.

11. These ideas are informed by Hunter, *Doctors' Stories*, 1991.

12. Riis, "Methodology," 2009.

13. See for example, Assimeng, *Saints*, 1986; Hertz, "St. Besse," [1913] 1983; Lemieux and Milot, ed. *Les croyances*, 1992; Milot, 'L'investigation," 1992; Orsi, "He Keeps Me Going," 1991; Orsi, *Thank You, Saint Jude*, 1994.

14. Brown, "Italian-Americans," 1999; Brown, "Saints," 1999; Carroll, *Cult of the Virgin Mary*, 1986; Carroll, *Catholic Cults*, 1989; Carroll, *Madonnas*, 1992; Iacovetta, *Such Hard-Working People*, 1992; Kraut, *Huddled Masses*, 1982, 120–121; Meagher, "Importance," 2008; Orsi, *The Madonna of 115th Street*, 1985; Stanger-Ross, *Staying Italian*, 2009; Varacalli et al., eds. *Saints in the Lives*, 1999; Zucchi, *Italians in Toronto*, 1988.

15. Boglioni and Lacroix, *Pèlerinages*, 1981; Lacroix, "Histoire," 1980; Lacroix and Boglioni, *Religions populaires*, 1972.

16. Cliche, *Les pratiques de devotion*, 1988.

17. Beaulieu and Beaulieu, *Pages d'histoire*, 1994; Ducharme, *Saint-Gabriel de Brandon*, 1917, 195–197.

18. Father Armand Gagné, Archiviste, Diocèse de Québec, personal communication, May 11, 2001.

19. George Minisci, interviews, January 18, 1995, February 2, 1995, September 26–27, 1996. The role of patrons in Italy and in immigrant committees is discussed in Gabaccia, *From Sicily to Elizabeth Street*, 1984, 50, 61, 105, 127.

20. Carroll, *Catholic Cults*, 1989, 57–78; Carroll, *Madonnas*, 1992, 115–120.

21. "Good Omen for World, Saint's Blood Liquifies," *Italy Daily*, Milan, September 22, 2001, http://www.freerepublic.com/focus/f-news/530283/posts, accessed June 30, 2010

22. Father F. J. Evans, interview, August 12, 1998.

23. "The Society's 'Humanitarian of the Year' Joe DeCandia," International Society of SS. Cosma & Damiano, *Eighth Annual Dinner Dance Program*, Howard Beach: Romaview Catering, 1998, np.

24. Stanger-Ross, *Staying Italian*, 2009, 69.

25. Clara told me her story in person, but it can now be read at the official website of the International Society of SS Cosma and Damiano, http://www.sscosmandamiano.com/aboutus.html, accessed October 31, 2012.

26. Dr. Geraldine M. Chapey, "A Tribute to Joe DeCandia," *The Wave, Rockaway's Newspaper*, May 2, 2003. http://www.rockawave.com/news/2003-05-02/Columnists/009.html, accessed October 31, 2012.

27. Cumbo, "Salvation in Indifference," 2001; Ferguson, *Women and Religion*, 1995, 142, 234–236; Jansen, *Italians*, 1988, 76; Orsi, *Thank You Saint Jude*, 1994.

28. Carroll, *American Catholics*, 80.

29. Anon., "Literary Notes," 1906; 5, Mercado, *Breve Historia*, 1985, 32, 36, 42–43; Muriel, *Hospitales . . . I*, 1956, 148–152, 243–245; Muriel, "Los hospitales," 1990, 240–241, 249; Muriel, *Hospitales . . . II*, 1991, 82, 103; Rodriguez, "Un espacio," 2006.

30. Ciudad Real, *Tratado curioso*, 1976, vol. 2, 195–219.

CHAPTER 4

1. David-Danel, "Les lieux de culte," 1966.

2. Vilarrasa i Coch, *Els Sants Metges*, 2004, 29–30, 41–59; Campabadal i Breu, "Vers una caracterització dels goigs," 2004.

3. From the events at Argelès-Sur-Mer website, http://es.argeles-sur-mer.com/, accessed October 31, 2012.

4. Müller, "Inventaire," 1893.

5. David-Danel, "Presence," 1986, 113; Pecker, *Médecine à Paris*, 1984, 18–22.

6. The Centre Catholique des Médecins Français maintains a website: http://frblin.perso.neuf.fr/ccmf/accueil.html, accessed October 31, 2012.

7. David-Danel, "Lieux de culte," 1966, 259, 260 (my translation); Gancel, *Saints qui guérissent*, vol. 1, 10–12; Renouard et Merrien, *Saints guérisseurs*, 1994.

8. Deichmann, *Ravenna*, 1989, vol. 2, pt. 2, 189, 322.

9. Wittmann, *Kosmas und Damian*, 1967, 32–39.

10. A translation of the Vatican manuscript dated 1101 is found in Pazzano and Capponi, *I santi medici*, 2000, 85–89.

11. Pazzano and Capponi, *I santi medici*, 2000, 99–100.

12. Russo, *Regesto Vaticano per la Calabria*, vol. 1, 1974, 58.

13. Wilstach, "Stone Beehive Homes," 1930.

14. Martellotta, *Memorie istoriche*, 1986. See also Morea, *Il culto*, [1886] 1996.

15. Cannito, *I santi medici*, 1998, 171.

16. Cannito, *I santi medici*, 1998, 179, 182.

17. Cannito, *I santi medici*, 1998, 234–246.

18. On ex-votos in general, see Cousin, *Ex-voto de Provence*, 1981; Cousin, *Le miracle et le quotidien*, 1983; Tripputi, *Bibliografia*, 1995, 11–64.

19. Cannito, *I santi medici*, 1998, 216, and figures between 216 and 217. On Bitonto's ex-voto paintings in context, see Angiuli, *Puglia ex voto*, 1977; Bronzini, *Santi e mercanti*, 1989.

20. More about the Foundation, its activities, and newsletter can be found on its website, http://www.santimedici.org/, accessed October 31, 2012.

21. Taviani-Carozzi, *La principauté lombarde de Salerne*, 1991, vol. 2, 800–828.

22. Ironically, the source for the earliest of medical practitioners in Salerno is a compendium of miracles attributed to Saint Trophimena, who was transplanted to the Salerno region by the Lombard conquest. Skinner, *Health and Medicine*, 1996, 41–42, 148–151; Taviani-Carozzi, *La principauté lombarde de Salerne*, 1991, vol. 2, 811–813.

23. Renzi, *Storia documentata*, 1857, 121–124, xxix–xxxii.

24. Carroll, *Catholic Cults*, 1989, 57–78; Carroll, *Madonnas*, 1992, 115–120.

25. Park and Park, "Saint Vitus' Dance," 1990.

26. Duffin, "Salerno, Saints, and Sutton's Law," 2009.

27. Martellotta, *Memorie istoriche*, 1986, 143n1.

28. Knight, *Discourse on the Worship of Priapus*, 1886, 17–23, esp. 18; Gioielli, *L'eremo dell'eros*, 2000.

29. Pazzano and Capponi, *I santi medici*, 2000, 115–116.

30. Darricau, "Une source," 1983.

31. Ditchfield, *Liturgy, Sanctity, and History*, 2002, 235 n. 93; Gentilcore, *Healers and Healing*, 1998, 177–202.

32. Menesto, *Il processo*, 1984; Park, *Secrets of Women*, 2006, 39–49.

33. Baldani, *I santi*, 2003; Frey, "Saints," 1979; Guest, *Healing Saints*, 2005, 81–94, 174–212; Lebrun, *Se soigner autrefois*, 1983, 113–116; Renouard and Merrien, *Saints guérisseurs*, 1994, 81–86; Théodoridès, "Saints," 1979.

34. Cahier, *Caracteristiques*, 1867, vol 2. 550–552; Chéreau, "Médecins béatifiés," 1874; Donzelli, *Calendario*, 1899; Frey, "Saints," 1979; Guest, *Healing Saints*, 2005, 70–75.

35. See for example, for Spain "Santos Medicos," http://idd0073h.eresmas.net/cam1bu4. htm; for Italy Associazione dei Consacrati/e Medici d'Italia, http://www.medicicon-sacrati.it/; for France, Amour et Vérité, Bioethique et Vie Humaine, Les saints médecins et litanie, http://www.amouretverite.org/. All accessed on October 31, 2012.

36. According to Martellotta, documentary evidence of the dates of origin of the most popular Italian celebrations of the santi medici are Oria (8thC), Isernia (1130), Matera (1230), Bitonto (14thC), Ravello (15thC), Anela (Sassari, 16thC), Napoli (1604), and Alberobello (1636). Elena (Gaeta) and Maglie (Lecce) also have important devotions

of great antiquity. Martellotta, *Memorie istoriche*, 1986, 143n1. To this list, we can add Riace (late 11thC). Pazzano and Capponi. *I santi medici*, 2000, 85–89.

37. Hickey, *Local Hospitals*, 1997, 134–174; Krueger, "Christian Piety," 2005; Risse, *Mending Bodies*, 1999, 91–106.

38. Temperini, *Basilica*, nd, 5.

CHAPTER 5

1. For example, Cullen, "Miracle," 1994; Fischer, "Nach der Taufe," 1999.

2. Wasserug, "It's a Miracle," 1989.

3. Debrousse and Duval, "Miracle ou mystère?" 1984.

4. Coppola, "Miracolo," 1999.

5. Brand and Yancey, "Miracle of Everyday Healing," 1985; Brett and Jersild, "Inappropriate Treatment," 2003; Connors and Smith, "Religious Insistence," 1996; Delisser, "Practical Approach," 2009; York, "Religious-Based Denial," 1987.

6. United States, *Subject Heading*, 1954.

7. See for example, Carrel, *Man*, 1935, 148–149; Carrel, *Voyage*, 1950; Composta, *Miracolo*, 1980; Leuret and Bon, *Modern Miraculous Cures*, 1957; Mangiapan, "Le contrôle médical," 1983; Sabourin, *Divine Miracles*, 1977, 151–172; Salleron, "Le miracle des evangiles," 1983; Szabo, "Seeing is Believing," 2002.

8. Mullin, *Miracles*, 1996, 40–46; Mullin, "Science, Miracles," 2003.

9. Gaudia, "About Intercessory Prayer," 2007.

10. Byrd, "Positive Therapeutic Effects," 1988.

11. See for example, Astin et al., "Efficacy," 2000; Sicher et al., "Randomized Double-Blind Study," 1998.

12. Matthews, "Religious Commitment," 1998; Matthews, "Prayer and Spirituality," 2000; Matthews et al., "Effects," 2000.

13. Roush, "Herbert Benson," 1997.

14. Dusek et al., "Study," 2002; Benson et al., "Study," 2006 ('excess of postoperative complications'); Koenig et al., "Religion, Spirituality and Medicine," 1999.

15. Puchalski and Larson, "Developing Curricula," 1998; Sloan, et al., "Religion, Spirituality, and Medicine," 1999; Sloan and Ramakrishnan, "Science, Medicine, and Intercessory Prayer," 2006.

16. Dusek et al., "Study," 2002.

17. Roberts et al., "Intercessory Prayer," 2000. See also Astin et al., "Efficacy," 2000.

18. Leibovici, "Effects of Remote, Retroactive Intercessory Prayer," 2001.

19. Hrobjartsson et al., "SILLY-bias," 2009.

20. Jorgensen, et al., "Divine Intervention?" 2009.

21. Hanson et al., "Providers," 2008.

22. Giacomini, "Theory-Based Medicine," 2009; Masters et al., "Demonstrable Effects?" 2006; Masters and Speilmans, "Prayer and Health," 2007.

23. Turner, "Just Another Drug?" 2006.

24. Hobbins, "Step," 2006.

25. Dennett, *Breaking the Spell*, 2006, 275–277.

26. Dworkin, *God Delusion*, 2006, 261–266.

27. Sloan and Ramakrishnan, "Science, Medicine, and Intercessory Prayer," 2006.

28. Hanson et al., "Providers," 2008.

29. On Brooklyn's *giglio*, see Brown, "Italian Americans," 1999; Carroll, *American Catholics*, 2007, 79; Sciorra, "We Go Where the Italians Live," 1999.

30. Duffin and Li, "Great Moments," 1995.

31. Orsi, "Religious Boundaires," 1999.

32. Bellande-Robertson, "Reading of Marassa Concept," 2006; Bellegarde-Smith, *Haiti: the Beached Citadel*, 1990, 9–22, 188–189; Brown, *Mama Lola*, 2001; Brown, "Afro-Caribbean Spirituality," 2006; Davis, *Serpent*, 1986, 72–73; Desmangles, *Faces of the Gods*, 1992; Drotbohm, *Geister*, 2005; Drotbohm, "Spirits and Virgins," 2008; Dubois, "Vodou and History," 2001; Hurbon, *Voodoo*, 1995, 82–83l; Louis, *Voodoo in Haiti*, 2007, 180–181.

33. Houlberg, "Magique Marassa," 1995 and 2005.

34. Wedel, *Santería Healing*, 2004, 181–182.

35. Patrick Bellegarde-Smith, personal communication, July 8, 2010.

36. Desmangeles, *Faces of the Gods*, 1992, 9; Drotbohm, *Geister*, 2005.

37. Drotbohm, "Spirits and Virgins," 2008, esp. 43.

38. Brown, *Mama Lola*, 2001, 247.

39. Bastide, Roger. "Le syncrétisme," 1965. My translation; another translation of "viol" is "rape."

40. Hurbon, *Voodoo*, 1995, 68.

41. Rey, "Catholic Pentecostalism," 2010.

42. Hess, "Domestic Medicine and Indigenous Medical Systems," 1984.

43. Christophe, *Rainbow*, 2006, 93–95; Desmangeles, *Faces of the Gods*, 1992, 7–8.

44. Julien, "Saints Côme et Damien," 1983; Shoemaker, "An Interview with William H. Helfand," 2011, 10.

45. Deren, *Divine Horsemen*, [1953] 1970, 38.

46. Mooney, *Faith Makes Us Live*, 2009, 243–247.

47. Yolette Toussaint, personal communication, September 26, 2010, and June 8, 2011.

48. Mooney, *Faith Makes Us Live*, 2009, 123 and 220.

49. Rey, "Ethnohistory of Haitian Pilgrimage," 2005. On medieval pilgrimage, see Scott, *Miracle Cures*, 2010.

50. On *goigs*, see Vilarrasa i Coch, *Els Sants Metges*, 2004, 97–163.

51. Graner, "From Osler with Love," 1996.

52. Gross, "Body Ritual," 1959; Dimsdale, "Nacirema Revisted," 2001.

53. Lee, "Evening Tea Break Ritual," 1999; Philpin, "Handing Over," 2006; Romanoff and Thompson, "Meaning Construction," 2006; Running et al. "Ritual," 2008; Wall, "Science and Ritual," 2003.

54. Sonnenberg, "Personal View," 2004.

55. Green, "Surgeons and Shamans," 2006; Peck et al. "Why Do We Keep Meeting Like This?" 2004.

CHAPTER 6

1. Melinsky, *Healing Miracles*, 1968, 73–110; Mullin, *Miracles and Magic*, 1979, 157–198; Mullin, *Miracles*, 1996, 83–104; O'Connell, "Roman Catholic Tradition," 1986; Peschel and Peschel, "Medical Miracles, 1988; Shaw, *Miracles in Enlightenment England*, 2006; Van Dam, *Saints and their Miracles*, 1993, 83–86; Vauchez, *Sainteté*, 1981, 544–558; Viguerie, "Les caractères permanents," 1983; Woodward, *Book of Miracles*, 2000, 368–369.
2. Larmer, *Water into Wine*, 1988, 83–92.
3. Hippocrates, "Sacred Disease," I.
4. Ferngren, *Medicine and Health Care*, 2009, 104–109; Risse, *Mending Bodies*, 1999, 77–78; Temkin, *Hippocrates*, 164, 183–183.
5. For studies on medieval and early modern coexistence of religion and medicine, Brockliss, "Medico-Religious Universe," 1989; see Dubois, "Les miracles," 1983; Sigal, *L'homme et le miracle*, 1985; Skinner, *Health and Medicine*, 1996; Vauchez, *Sainteté*, 1981.
6. Huth and Murray, *Medicine in Quotations*, 2000, 129, 281.
7. Mullin, "Science, Miracles," 2003, 205; Shaw, *Miracles in Enlightenment England*, 2006, 1–3, 21–33; Trenard, "Les miracles ralliés par Voltaire," 1983.
8. Anon., "Miracles (de *La Lancette Belge*)," 1880.
9. For a medical practitioner's definition that requires an understanding of God, see Sulmasy, "What is a Miracle?" 2007.
10. Overall, "Miracles as Evidence," 1985.
11. Williams, *Idea of the Miraculous*, 1990, 137–157, esp. 157.
12. Corner, *Signs of God*, 2005, 198; Swinburne, *Concept of Miracle*, 1970, 71.
13. Cotter, *Miracles*, 1999, 185–178.
14. Amundsen and Ferngren, "Early Christian Tradition," 1986; Ferngren, *Medicine and Health Care*, 2009, 62–63, 104–109; Temkin, *Hippocrates*, 1991, 126–138, 213–216; Wallis, "Experience of the Book," 1995, 117–124.
15. See for example, Berland, "Can the Self Affect the Course of Cancer," 1995; Romanoff and Thompson, "Meaning Construction," 2006; Scott, *Miracle Cures*, 2010.

EPILOGUE

1. Margaret Wente, "On a Pill and a Prayer," *Globe and Mail*, October 23, 2010.
2. André Picard, "Do 'Medical Miracles' Really Exist?" *Globe and Mail*, October 20, 2010.

Bibliography

Adam of Bremen. *History of the Archbishops of Hamburg-Bremen*, ed. Francis Joseph Tschan. New York: Columbia University Press, 1959.

Adnès, André, and Pierre Canivet. "Guérisons miraculeuses et exorcismes dans "l'Histoire Philothé" de Theodoret de Cyr." *Revue de l'histoire des religions* 171 (1967): 53–82, 149–179.

Albert, Maurice. *Le culte de Castor et Pollux en Italie*. Paris: Thorin, 1882.

Amundsen, Darrel W. "The Medieval Christian Tradition." In *Caring and Curing. Health and Medicine in the Western Religious Traditions*, ed. Ronald L. Numbers and Darrel W. Amundsen, 65–107. New York and London: Macmillan, 1986.

———. *Medicine, Society, and Faith in the Ancient and Medieval Worlds*. Baltimore: Johns Hopkins University Press, 1996.

Amundsen, Darrel W., and Gary B. Ferngren. "The Early Christian Tradition." In *Caring and Curing. Health and Medicine in the Western Religious Traditions*, ed. Ronald L. Numbers and Darrel W. Amundsen, 40–60. New York and London: Macmillan, 1986.

Angenendt, Arnold. *Heilige und Reliquien: die Geschichte ihres kultes com fruhen Christentum bis zur Gegenvart*. Munchen: C. H. Beck, 1994.

Angiuli, Emanuela, ed. *Puglia ex Voto; Barí, Biblioteca Provinciale de Gemmis, 1977*. Lecce: Congedo Editore, 1977.

Anonymous. "Literary Notes." *British Medical Journal* (1906): 1876.

———. "Miracles (de *La Lancette Belge*) [editorial]." *Union médical du Canada* 9 (1880): 144.

———. "Grey Nuns Founder Canonized. Quebec Widow Becomes First Catholic Saint Born in Canada." *Globe and Mail*, 10 December 1990, A1.

Assimeng, Max. *Saints and Social Structures*. Tema, Ghana: Ghana Publishing, 1986.

Astin, John A., Elaine Harkness, and Edzard Ernst. "The Efficacy of 'Distant Healing'; A Systematic Review of Randomized Trials." *Annals of Internal Medicine* 132, no. 11 (2000): 903–910.

Bagnell, Kenneth. *Canadese. A Portrait of the Italian Canadians*. Toronto: Macmillan, 1989.

Baldani, Paolo. *I santi che guariscono*. Casale Monferrato: Piemme, 2003.

Ball, Warwick. *Rome in the East: the Transformation of an Empire*. London: Routledge, 2000.

Baring-Gould, S. "SS Cosmas and Damian." In *The Lives of the Saints*, 397–401. Edinburgh: John Grant, 1914.

Barkan, Leonard. "Cosmas and Damian: of Medicine, Miracles and the Economies of the Body." In *Organ Transplantation: Meanings and Realities*, ed. Stuart J. Younger, Renée C. Fox, and Laurence J. O'Connell, 221–251. Madison: University of Wisconsin Press, 1996.

Bastide, Roger. "Le syncrétisme en Amérique Latine." *Bulletin Saint Jean-Baptiste* 5 (1965): 166–71; also online at Bastidiana, 43–44 (2003), http://claude.ravelet. pagesperso-orange.fr/syncrétisme.pdf, accessed October 31, 2012.

Beaulieu, Maurice, and Thérèse Beaulieu. *Pages d'histoire de St Damien-de-Brandon*. St Gabriel-de-Brandon: T. Beaulieu, 1994.

Beit-Hallahmi, Benjamin, and Maria Paluszny. "Twinship in Mythology and Science: Ambivalence, Differentiation, and the Magical Bond." *Comprehensive Psychiatry* 15, no. 4 (1974): 345–353.

Bellande-Robertson, Florence. "A Reading of the Marasa Concept in Lilas Desquiron's *Les Chemins de Loco-Miroir*." In *Haitian Vodou: Spirit, Myth, Reality*, ed. Patrick Bellegarde-Smith and Claudine Michel. Bloomington: Indiana University Press, 2006.

Bellegarde-Smith, Patrick. *Haiti: The Beached Citadel*. Boulder, San Francisco, and London: Westview Press, 1990.

Benson, Herbert, J.A. Dusek, Jane B. Sherwood, Peter Lam, Charles F. Bethea, William Carpenter, Sidney Levitsky, Peter C. Hill, Donald W. Clem, Manoj K. Jain, David Drummel, Stephen L. Kopecky, Paul S. Mueller, Dean Marke, Sue Rollins, and Patricia Hibberd. "Study of the Therapeutic Effects of Intercessory Prayer (STEP) in Cardiac Bypass Patients: A Multicenter Randomized Trial of Uncertainty and Certainty of Receiving Intercessory Prayer." *American Heart Journal* 151, no. 4 (2006): 934–942.

Berland, Warren. "Can the Self Affect the Course of Cancer: Unexpected Cancer Recovery: Why Patients Believe They Survive." *Advances; The Journal of Mind Body Health* 11, no. 4 (1995): 5–19.

Boglioni, Pierre, and Benoît Lacroix. *Les pèlerinages au Québec*. Québec: Les Presses de l'Université Laval, 1981.

Boobyer, G. H. "The Gospel Miracles: Views Past and Present." In *The Miracles and the Resurrection; Some Recent Studies*, ed. Ian T. Ramsey, G.H. Boobyer, F. N. Davey, M. C. Perry, and Henry Cadbury, J., 31–49. London: S.P.C.K.; Theological Collections no. 3, 1964.

Borella, Jean. *Le mystère du signe: histoire et théories du symbole. Collection Métalangage*. Paris: Editions Maisonneuve et la Rose, 1989.

Brand, P., and P. Yancey. "The Miracle of Everyday Healing: Expecting the Extraordinary Can Be Dangerous." *Journal of Christian Nursing* 2, no. 2 (1985): 4–8.

Brett, Allan S., and Paul Jersild. "'Inappropriate' Treatment near the End of Life: Conflict between Religious Convictions and Clinical Judgment." *Archives of Internal Medicine* 163, no. 14 (2003): 1645–1649.

Brockliss, L. W. B. "The Medico-Religious Universe of an Early Eighteenth-Century Parisian Doctor: the Case of Philippe Hecquet." In *The Medical Revolution of the Seventeenth Century*, ed. Roger French and Andrew Wear, 191–221. Cambridge: Cambridge University Press, 1989.

Bronzini, Giovanni Battista. "Santi e mercanti sui mari de Puglia." *Lares* LV, no. n. 1 (1989): 5–35.

Brown, Karen McCarthy. *Mama Lola: a Vodou Priestess in Brooklyn*. 2nd ed. Berkeley: University of California Press, 2001.

———. "Afro-Caribbean Spirituality: A Haitian Case Study." In *Invisible Powers: Vodou in Haitian Life and Culture*, ed. Claudine Michel and Patrick Bellegarde-Smith, 1–26. New York: Palgrave Macmillan, 2006.

Brown, Mary Elizabeth. "Italian-Americans and Their Saints: Historical Considerations." In *The Saints in the Lives of Italian-Americans: An Interdisciplinary Investigation*, ed. Joseph A. Varacalli, Salvatore Primeggia, Salvatore LaGumina, and Donald J. D'Elia, 35–67. Stony Brook, NY: Forum Italicum, Supplement, Filibary No. 14, 1999.

———. "The Saints in the Lives of Italian Americans: A Bibliographic Essay." In *The Saints in the Lives of Italian-Americans: An Interdisciplinary Investigation*, ed. Joseph A. Varacalli, Salvatore Primeggia, Salvatore LaGumina, and Donald J. D'Elia, 264–281. Stony Brook, NY: Forum Italicum, Supplement, Filibary No. 14, 1999.

Brown, P. R. L. "Aspects of the Christianization of the Roman Aristocracy." *Journal of Roman Studies* 51 (1961): 2–11.

———. *The Cult of the Saints: Its Rise and Function in Latin Christianity*. Chicago: University of Chicago Press, 1981.

Byrd, Randolph C. "Positive Therapeutic Effects of Intercessory Prayer in a Coronary Care Unit Population." *Southern Medical Journal* 8, no. 7 (1988): 826–829.

Cahier, Charles. *Caractéristiques des saints dans l'art populaire*. 2 vols. Paris: Poussielgue, 1867.

Campabadal i Breu, Joan. "Vers una caracterització dels goigs. Un cas concret: Sant Cosme i Sant Damià." In *Els Sants Metges guaridors, Sant Cosme i Sant Damià: història, llegenda i goigs*, ed. Josep M Vilarrasa i Coch, 97–163. Barcelona: Editorial Mediterrània, 2004.

Canguilhem, Georges. "Histoire des religions et histoire des sciences." In *Mélanges Alexandre Koyré*, 69–87. Paris: Hermann, 1964.

Cannito, Giuseppe. *I santi medici Cosma e Damiano nella storia e nel culto. Note storiche in Bitonto*. Bitonto: Edizioni Basilica Santuario, 1998.

Caraffa, F. *San Cosimato: l'abbazia e la chiesa di Mica Aurea in Trastevere, Monographie Romane*. Roma: Alma Roma, 1971.

Carpenter, Edward. *Pagan and Christian Creeds: Their Origin and Meaning*. New York: Harcourt Brace and Company, 1971.

Carrel, Alexis. *Man the Unknown*. New York and London: Harper, 1935.

———. *The Voyage to Lourdes*. Trans. Virgilia Peterson. New York: Harper, 1950.

Carroll, Michael P. *The Cult of the Virgin Mary: Psychological Origins*. Princeton: Princeton University Press, 1986.

———. *Catholic Cults and Devotions: A Psychological Inquiry*. Montreal and Kingston: McGill Queen's University Press, 1989.

———. *Madonnas that Maim: Popular Catholicism in Italy since the Fifteenth Century*. Baltimore and London: Johns Hopkins University Press, 1992.

———. *American Catholics in the Protestant Imagination: Rethinking the Academic Study of Religion*. Baltimore: Johns Hopkins University Press, 2007.

Chéreau, A. "Médecins béatifiés." In *Dictionnaire encyclopédique des sciences médicale*, ed. Amédée Dechambre, 727–729. Paris: Masson et fils, 1874.

Christophe, Marc A. "Rainbow over Water: Haitian Art, Vodou Aetheticism, and Philosophy." In *Haitian Vodou: Spirit, Myth, and Reality*, ed. Patrick Bellegarde-Smith and Claudine Michel, 84–102. Bloomington, Indiana University Press, 2006.

Cimino, Stephen F. *St. Anthony of Padua, 75th Anniversary Edition*. Utica, N.Y.: St. Anthony of Padua Church, 1987.

Ciudad Real, Antonio de. *Tratado curioso y docto de las grandezas de la Nueva España*. Ed. Josefina García Quintana and Victo M. Castillo Farreras. 2 vols. Mexico: Universidad Nacional Autónoma de Mexico, 1976.

Cliche, Marie-Aimée. *Les pratiques de dévotion en Nouvelle-France: comportements populaires et encadrement ecclésial dans le gouvernement de Québec*. Québec, Presses de l'Université Laval, 1988.

Composta, Dario. *Il miracolo: realta o suggestione? Rassegna documentata di fatti staordinari nel cinquentennio, 1920–1970*. Rome: Città Nuova Editrice, 1981.

Congregatio pro causis sanctorum. *Marianopolitana. Canonizationis . . . Mariae Margaritae Dufrost de Lajemmerais (viduae Youville). Positio super miraculo*. Rome: Guerra, 1989.

Connors, R. B., and M. L. Smith. "Religious Insistence on Medical Treatment: Christian Theology and Re-Imagination." *Hastings Center Report* 26, no. 4 (1996): 23–30.

Coppola, Vincenzo. "Il miraculo della radiologia. Riflessioni sul un caso di guarigione inspiegabile commentata con al diagnostica per immagini." *Radiologica Medica* 98, no. 4 (1999): 225–229.

Cotter, Wendy. *Miracles in Greco-Roman Antiquity: a Sourcebook*. London: Routledge, 1999.

Corner, Mark. *Signs of God: Miracles and Their Interpretation*. Aldershot: Ashgate, 2005.

Cousin, Bernard. *Ex-voto de Provence: Images de la religion populaire et de la vie d'autrefois*. Bruges: Desclée de Brouwer, 1981.

———. *Le miracle et le quotidien. Les ex voto en Provence, images d'une société.* Aix-en-Provence: CNRS, Sociétés Mentalités Cultures, 1983.

Csepregi, Ildikó. "Mysteries for the Uninitiated: The Role and Symbolism of the Eucharist in Miraculous Dream Healing." In *The Eucharist in Theology and Philosophy: Issues of Doctrinal History in East and West from the Patristic Age to the Reformation,* ed. István Perczei, 97–130. Leuven: Leuven University Press, 2005.

Cullen, Johanna C. "The Miracle of Bolsena: Growth of Serratia on Sacramental Bread and Polenta May Explain Incidents in Medieval Italy." *ASM News* 60, no. April (1994): 187–191.

Cumbo, Enrico Carlson. "Salvation in Indifference: Gendered Expressions of Italian-Canadian Immigrant Catholicity, 1900–1940." In *Households of Faith: Family, Gender and Community in Canada, 1760–1969,* ed. Nancy Christie, 205–233. Montreal: McGill-Queen's University Press, 2001.

Darricau, Raymond. "Une source sur l'histoire des miracles: 'positio super miraculis.'" In *Histoire des miracles. Actes de la Sixième Rencontre d'Histoire Religieuse, 8–9 octobre 1982,* ed. Jean de Viguerie, 165–172. Angers: Presses de l'Université d'Angers, 1983.

Dasen, Véronique. *Jumeaux, jumelles, dans l'antiquité grecque et romaine.* Zurich: Akanthus Verlag für Archäologie, 2005.

David-Danel, Marie-Louise. *Iconographie des saints médecins Côme et Damien.* Lille: Université de Lille and Morel et Corduant, 1958.

———. "Les lieux de culte des saints Côme et Damien en France." In *Mélanges Joseph Coppin, littérature et religion, Mélanges de science religieuse,* 23 supplement (1966); 251–262.

———. *Répertoire pour la France des lieux de culte dédiés aux saints Côme et Damien* [collection of 4 reprints from *Mélanges des Sciences Religieuses, 1966–1969*], ca 1969.

———. "Saint-Côme et Saint Damien patrons des pharmaciens." In *Saint Côme et Saint Damien. Culte et iconographie,* ed. Pierre Julien and François Ledermann, 23–28. Zurich: Juris Druck, 1985.

———. "Presence de Côme et Damien à Luzarches." *Revue d'histoire de la pharmacie* 74, no. 270 (1986): 203–206.

Davis, Wade. *The Serpent and the Rainbow.* Toronto: Stoddart Press, 1986.

De Simoni, Emilia, ed. *Ex voto tra storia e antropologia.* Rome: De Luca Editore, 1986.

Debrousse, J.-Y., and R. Duval. "Un miracle ou un mystère? A propos de guerison spontanée tardive." *Bulletin de la Société d'Ophthalmologistes de France* 84, no. 12 (1984): 1451–1453.

Deichmann, Friedrich Wilhelm. *Ravenna, Hauptstadt des Spätantiken Abendlandes.* 3 vols. Stuttgart: Franz Steiner, 1989.

Delehaye, Hippolyte. "Castor et Pollux dans les légendes hagiographiques (essay review)." *Analecta Bollandiana* XXIII (1904): 427–432.

———. "Recueil antique de miracles des saints." *Analecta Bollandiana* XLIII (1925): 5–85, 305–325.

——. *The Legends of the Saints*. Trans. Donald Attwater. New York: Fordham University Press, 1962.

Delisser, Horace M. "A Practical Approach to the Family that Expects a Miracle." *Chest* 135, no. 6 (2009): 1643–1647.

Dennett, Daniel. *Breaking the Spell: Religion as a Natural Phenomenon*. New York: Viking, 2006.

Deren, Maya. *Divine Horsemen: Voodoo Gods of Haiti*. London, Thames and Hudson, [1953] 1970.

Desmangles, Leslie G. *The Faces of the Gods: Vodou and Roman Catholicism in Haïti*. Chapel Hill and London: University of North Carolina Press, 1992.

Deubner, Ludwig. *Kosmas und Damian. Texte und Einleitung*. Leipzig; Aalen: Scienta Verlag, [1907] 1980.

Dimsdale, Joel E. "The Nacirema Revisited." *Annals of Behavioral Medicine* 23, no. 1 (2001): 75–76.

Ditchfield, Simon. *Liturgy, Sanctity, and History in Tridentine Italy: Pietro Maria Campi and the Preservation of the Particular*. Cambridge: Cambridge University Press, 2002.

Donzelli, Giuseppe. *Il calendario dei santi medici compilato nel 1667*. Napoli: Pierro e Veraldi, 1899.

Drotbohm, Heike. *Geister in der Diaspora. Haitianische Diskurse über Geschlechter, Jugend und Macht in Montreal, Kanada ['Spirits in the diaspora. Haitian discourses on gender, youth and power in Montreal, Canada']*. Marburg: Curupira, 2005.

——. "Of Spirits and Virgins: Situating Belonging in Haitian Religious Spaces in Montreal, Canada." *Suomen Anthropologi. Journal of the Finnish Anthropological Society* 33, no. 1 (2008): 33–50.

——. "Haunted by Spirits: Balancing Religious Commitment and Moral Obligations in Haitian Transnational Social Fields." In *Traveling Spirits: Migrants, Markets and Mobilities*, ed. Gertrud Hüwelmeier and Kristine Krause, 36–51. Abingdon, Oxon, and New York: Routledge, 2010.

Dubois, Elfrieda. "Les miracles et les reformes en Angleterre aux seizième et dix-septième siècles." In *Histoire des miracles. Actes de la Sixième Rencontre d'Histoire Religieuse, 8–9 octobre 1982*, ed. Centre de recherches d'histoire religieuse et d'histoire des idées Université d'Angers, 51–61. Angers: Presses de l'Université d'Angers, 1983.

Dubois, Laurent. "Vodou and History." *Comparative Studies in Society and History* 43, no.1 (2001): 92–100.

Ducharme, Gabriel. *Histoire de Saint-Gabriel de Brandon et de ses démembrements*. Montreal, G. Ducharme, 1917.

Duffin, Jacalyn. *Medical Miracles; Doctors, Saints, and Healing in the Modern World*. New York: Oxford University Press, 2009.

——. "Salerno, Saints, and Sutton's Law: On the Origin of Europe's 'First' Medical School." *Medical Hypotheses* 73 (2009): 265–267.

Duffin, Jacalyn, and Alison Li. "Great Moments: Parke, Davis & Co, and the Creation of Medical Art." *Isis* 86, no. 1–29 (1995).

Durkheim, Emile. "Concerning the Definition of Religious Phenomena [1899]." In *Durkheim on Religion*, ed. W.S.F. Pickering, 74–99. London and Boston: Routledge and Kegan Paul, 1975.

———. *The Elementary Forms of Religious Life*. Trans. Joseph Ward Swain. New York: The Free Press, [1915] 1965.

Dusek, Jeffery A., Jane B. Sherwood, Richard Friedman, Patricia Myers, Charles F. Bethea, Sidney Levitsky, Peter C. Hill, Manoj K. Jain, Stephen L. Kopecky, Paul S. Mueller, Peter Lam, Herbert Benson, and Patricia L. Hibberd. "Study of the Therapeutic Effects of Intercessory Prayer (STEP): Study Design and Research Methods." *American Heart Journal* 143, no. 4 (2002): 577–584.

Dworkin, Richard. *The God Delusion*. Boston and New York: Houghton Mifflin, 2006.

Eamon, William. "Technology as Magic in the Late Middle Ages and the Renaissance." *Janus* 70 (1983): 171–203.

Eisenbichler, Konrad, ed. *An Italian Region in Canada: the Case of Friuli-Venezia Giulia*. Toronto: Multicultural History Society of Ontario, 1998.

Evensen, Stein A., and Per Stavem. "Long-Term Survival in Acute Leukemia." *Acta Medica Scandinavica* 219, no. 1 (1986): 79–83.

Ferguson, Marianne. *Women and Religion*. Englewood Cliffs, N.J.: Prentice Hall, 1995.

Ferland-Angers, Albertine. *Mère d'Youville: Vénérable Marie-Marguerite du Frost de Lajemmerais Veuve d'Youville 1701–1771*. Montreal: Librairie Beauchemin, 1945.

Ferngren, Gary B. "Early Christianity as a Religion of Healing." *Bulletin of the History of Medicine* 66 (1992): 1–15.

———. *Medicine and Health Care in Early Christianity*. Baltimore: Johns Hopkins University Press, 2009.

Festugière, André Jean. *Vie de Theodore de Sykeôn*. Bruxelles, Société des Bollandistes, 1970.

———, ed. *Sainte Thècle, Saints Côme et Damien, Saints Cyr et Jean, Saint Georges (extraits)*. Paris: A. et J. Picard, 1971.

Fischer, C. "Nach der Taufe erschien ein rotes Kreuz auf der Stirn. Kein Wunder—nur phototoxische Reaktion auf Duftessenz. [After baptism a red cross appeared on the forehead. Not a miracle—only a phototoxic reaction to perfume essence]." *MMW Fortschritte der Medizin* 141, no. 47 (1999): 44.

Frey, Emil F. "Saints in Medical History." *Clio Medica* 14 (1979): 35–70.

Frézouls, Edmond. "Recherches historiques et archéologiques sur la ville de Cyrrhus." *Les Annales archéologiques de Syrie* IV-V (1954–55): 89–128.

Gabaccia, Donna R. *From Sicily to Elizabeth Street: Housing and Social Change Among Italian Immigrants*. Albany, NY: State University of New York, 1984.

Gale, R. P., and K. A. Foon. "Acute Myeloid Leukemia: Recent Advances in Therapy." *Clinics in Hematology* 15, no. 3 (1986): 781–810.

Gancel, Hippolyte. *Les saints qui guérissent en Bretagne.* 2 vols. Rennes: Editions France Ouest, 2000.

Gärtner, Bertil. *The Theology of the Gospel of Thomas.* London: Collins, 1961.

Gaudia, Gil. "About Intercessory Prayer: the Scientific Study of Miracles" *Medgenmed: Medscape General Medicine* 9, no. 1 (2007): 56.

Gedda, Luigi. *Twins in History and Science.* Trans. Marco Milani-Comparetti. Springfield IL: Charles C. Thomas, 1961.

Gentilcore, David. *Healers and Healing in Early Modern Italy.* Manchester: Manchester University Press, 1998.

Giacomini, Mita. "Theory-Based Medicine and the Role of Evidence: Why the Emperor Needs New Clothes, Again." *Perspectives in Biology & Medicine* 52, no. 2 (2009): 234–251.

Giannarelli, Elena, ed. *Cosma e Damiano dall'Oriente a Firenze.* Firenze: Edizione della Meridiana, 2002.

Gioielli, Mauro. *L'eremo dell'eros: La festa dei santi Cosma e Damiano a Isernia.* Campobasso: Palladino, 2000.

Ginzburg, Carlo. *The Cheese and the Worms. The Cosmos of a Sixteenth-Century Miller.* Trans. John and Anne Tedeschi. Baltimore and London: Johns Hopkins University Press, 1980.

Goodich, Michael. *Lives and Miracles of the Saints: Studies in Medieval Latin Hagiography.* Aldershot, Hants, England; Burlington, VT: Ashgate/Variorum, 2004.

Graner, John L. "From Osler with Love: the Mayo Brothers' Cosmas and Damian Print." *Mayo Clinic Proceedings* 71, no. 7 (1996): 717–718.

Grant, Michael. *The Roman Forum.* London: Weidenfeld and Nicolson, 1970.

Green, Stephen A. "Surgeons and Shamans: the Placebo Value of Ritual." *Clinical Orthopaedics and Related Research* 450 (2006): 249–254.

Gross, P. A. "Body Ritual among the Nacirema: a Note on Medical Anthropology and Magic in Medicine." *New England Journal of Medicine* 261 (1959): 757–758.

Guest, R. Gerald. *The Healing Saints of Medicine.* Markham, Ontario: Arma Dei, 2005.

Hamilton, Mary. *Incubation, or the Cure of Disease in Pagan Temples and Christian Churches.* London and St. Andrews: Simpkin, Marshall, Hamilton, Kent, Co. and W.C. Henderson, 1906.

Hankoff, Leon D. "Why the Healing Gods are Twins." *Yale Journal of Biology and Medicine* 50 (1977): 307–319.

Hanson, Laura C., Debra Dobbs, Barbara M. Usher, Sharon Williams, Jim Rawlings, and Timothy P. Daaleman. "Providers and Types of Spiritual Care During Serious Illness." *Journal of Palliative Medicine* 11, no. 6 (2008): 907–914.

Hardon, John A. "Concept of Miracle from Saint Augustine to Modern Apologetics." *Theological Studies* XV (1954): 229–257.

Harney, Robert F. "Toronto's Little Italy." In *Little Italies in North America,* ed. Robert F. Harney and J. Vincenza Scarpaci, 41–62. Toronto: Multicultural History Society of Ontario, 1981.

Harris, J. Rendel. *The Dioscuri in Christian Legends*. London: C.J. Clay and Cambridge University Press, 1903.

Harrison, Peter. "Miracles, Early Modern Science and Rational Religion." *Church History* 75, no. 3 (2006): 493–510.

Hart, Gerald D. *Asclepius: The God of Medicine*. London: Royal Society of Medicine Press, 2000.

Hertz, Robert. "St Besse: Study of an Alpine Cult [1913]." In *Saints and Their Cults; Studies in Religious Sociology, Folklore, and History*, ed. Stephen Wilson, 55–100. Cambridge, London, New York, New Rochelle, Melbourne, Sydney: Cambridge University Press, 1983.

Hess, Salinda. "Domestic Medicine and Indigenous Medical Systems in Haiti: Culture and Political Economy of Health in a Disemic Society." PhD thesis, Anthropology. McGill University, Montreal, 1984.

Hickey, Daniel. *Local Hospitals and Ancien Régime France: Rationalization, Resistance, Renewal, 1530–1789*. Montreal and Kingston: McGill-Queen's University Press, 1997.

Higgins, Michael W. *Stalking the Holy: The Pursuit of Saint-Making*. Toronto: Anansi, 2006.

Hippocrates. "The Sacred Disease." In *Hippocrates with an English Translation*. Vol. 2, ed. W. H. S. Jones, 139–183. London: Heinemann; Loeb Classical Library 148, 1923.

Hobbins, Peter. "A Step Towards More Ethical Prayer Studies." *American Heart Journal* 152, no. 4 (2006): e33.

Holmes, Megan. *Fra Filippo Lippi the Carmelite Painter*. New Haven: Yale University Press, 1999.

Horden, Peregrine. "Saints and Doctors in the Early Byzantine Empire: The Case of Theodore of Sykeon." In *The Church and Healing. Studies in Church History Vol. 19*, ed. W. J. Sheils, 1–13. Oxford: B. Blackwell for the Ecclesiatical History Society, 1982.

Houlberg, Marilyn. "Magique Marasa: The Ritual Cosmos of Twins and Other Sacred Children." In *Sacred Arts of Haitian Vodou*, ed. Donald J. Consentino, 267–283. Los Angeles: UCLA Fowler Museum of Cultural History, 1995.

———. "Magique Marasa: The Ritual Cosmos of the Twins and Other Sacred Children." In *Fragments of Bone: Neo-African Religions in a New World*, ed. Patrick Bellegarde-Smith, 13–31: University of Illinois Press, 2005.

Houston, John. *Reported Miracles: A Critique of Hume*. Cambridge: Cambridge University Press, 1994.

Hrobjartsson, Asbjorn, Karsten J. Jorgensen, and Ulrik A. Felding. "En ny videnskabelig fejlkilde: SILLY-bias. Analyse af citationer af BMJ's juleartikler. [A new scientific source of bias: SILLY bias. Analysis of citations of BMJ's Christmas articles]." *Ugeskrift for Laeger* 171, no. 51 (2009): 3784–3789.

Huisman, Frank G. "Human Frailty versus God's Omnipotence: The Meaning of the Miracle of the Black Leg." In *One Leg in the Grave; The Miracle of the Transplantation of the Black Leg*, ed. Kees W. Zimmerman, 43–62. Maarsen: Elsevier/Bunge, 1998.

Hunter, Kathryn Montgomery. *Doctors' Stories: The Narrative Structure of Medical Knowledge*. Princeton, N.J.: Princeton University Press, 1991.

Hurbon, Laennec. *Voodoo: Search for the Spirit*. New York: Harry N. Abrams, 1995.

Huth, Edward, and T. Jock Murray. *Medicine in Quotations: Views of Health and Disease through the Ages*. Philadelphia: American College of Physicians, 2000.

Iacovetta, Franca. *Such Hardworking People: Italian Immigrants in Post-War Toronto*. Montreal and Kingston: McGill-Queen's University Press, 1992.

Jackson, Ralph. *Doctors and Diseases in the Roman Empire*. Norman and London: University of Oklahoma Press, 1988.

Jansen, Clifford J. *Factbook on Italians in Canada*. Toronto: Department of Sociology York University, 1987.

———. *Italians in a Multicultural Canada*, Canadian Studies Series vol. 1. Lewiston and Queenston: Edwin Mellen Press, 1988.

Jones, Prudence, and Nigel Pennick. *A History of Pagan Europe*. London: Routledge, 1995.

Jorgensen, Karsten Juhl, Asbjorn Hrobjartsson, and Peter C. Gotzsche. "Divine Intervention? A Cochrane Review on Intercessory Prayer Gone Beyond Science and Reason." *Journal of Negative Results in Biomedicine* 8, no. 7 (2009).

Judson, Katherine B. *Native Legends of the Great Lakes and the Mississippi Valley*. DeKalb, Ill.: Northern Illinois University Press, 2000.

Julien, Pierre. "Un sanctuaire lyonnais dédié aux saints Côme et Damien." *Revue d'histoire de la pharmacie* 20, no. Dec. (1970): 243–251.

———. "La confrérie des Saints Côme et Damien à Luzarches." *Revue d'histoire de la pharmacie* 21 (1973): 505–518.

———. *Saint Côme et Saint Damien, patrons des médecins, chirurgiens, et pharmaciens*. Paris: Louis Pariente, 1980.

———. "Le point sur les ex libris professionels à l'effigie des saints Côme et Damien." *Revue d'histoire de la pharmacie* 29 (1982): 176–178.

———. "Les Saints Côme et Damien aux Pay-Bas, en Sicile, et de l'Afrique, à Haïti, et au Brésil." *Revue d'histoire de la pharmacie* 71, no. 256 (1983): 77–79.

———. "Côme et Damien, hier et aujourd'hui. Quelques questions." In *Saint Côme et Saint Damien. Culte et iconographie*, ed. Pierre Julien and François Ledermann, 43–62. Zurich: Juris Druck, 1985.

Julien, Pierre, and François Ledermann, ed. *Saint Côme et Saint Damien. Culte et iconographie*, Colloque, Mendriso, September 29–30, 1985. Zurich: Juris Druck & Verlag, 1985.

Julien, Pierre, François Ledermann, and Alain Touwaide. *Cosma e Damiano dal culto populare alle protezione di chirurghi, medici, e farmacisti: aspetti e immagini*. Milan: Antea Edizioni, 1993.

Kahan, Barry D. "Cosmas and Damian Revisited." *Transplantation Proceedings* Supplement 1 (1983): 2211–2216.

Kazhdan, A., ed. *Oxford Dictionary of Byzantium*. New York and Oxford, Oxford University Press, 1991.

Keating, Michael J., Kenneth B. McCredie, Gerald P. Bodey, Terry L. Smith, Edmund Gehan, and Emil J. Freireich. "Improved Prospects for Long-Term Survival in Adults with Acute Myelogenous Leukemia." *JAMA* 248, no. 19 (1982): 2481–2486.

Kee, Howard Clark. *Medicine, Miracle, and Magic in New Testament Times*. Cambridge: Cambridge University Press, 1986.

Keller, Ernst, and Marie-Luise Keller. *Miracles in Dispute. A Continuing Debate*. London: SCM Press Ltd, 1969.

Knight, Richard P. *A Discourse on the Worship of Priapus and Its Connections to the Mystic Theology of the Ancients*. London: T. Spilsbury, 1886.

Koenig, Harold G., Ellen Idler, Stanislav Kasl, Judith C. Hays, Linda K. George, Marc Musick, David B. Larson, Terence R. Collins, Herbert Benson. "Religion, Spirituality and Medicine: A Rebuttal to the Skeptics." *International Journal of Psychiatry and Medicine* 29 (1999): 123–131.

Krappe, Alexander Haggerty. *Mythologie universelle*. New York: Arno Press, [1930] 1978.

Kraut, Alan M. *The Huddled Masses: the Immigrant in American Society, 1880–1921*. Arlington Heights, Ill.: Harlan Davidson, 1982.

Kroeber, Karl, ed. *Native American Storytelling*. Oxford: Blackwell, 2004.

Krueger, Derek. "Christian Piety and Practice in the Sixth Century." In *The Cambridge Companion to the Age of Justinian*, ed. Michael Maas, 291–315. Cambridge: Cambridge University Press, 2005.

Labriola, P. Angelo. *I Santi Cosma e Damiano: medici e martiri*. Roma: Ed. Analecta T.O.R., 1984.

Lacroix, Benoit. "Histoire et religion traditionelle des Québécois (1534–1970)." In *Culture populaire et littératures au Québec*, ed. René Bouchard. Saratoga, Calif.: Anima Libri, 1980.

Lacroix, Benoit, and Pietro Boglioni, ed. *Les religions populaires. Colloque international, 1970*. Québec: Presses de l'Université Laval. Histoire et Sociologie de la Culture no. 3, 1972.

Lambertini, Prospero (Benedict XIV). *De servorum Dei beatificatione et beatorum canonizatione . . .* 4 vols. Bononiae (Bologna): Formis Longhi, 1734–1738.

Larmer, Robert A. H. *Water into Wine: An Investigation of the Concept of Miracle*. Kingston and Montreal: McGill-Queen's University Press, 1988.

———, ed. *Questions of Miracle*. Montreal and Kingston: McGill-Queen's University Press, 1996.

Larson, Gerald James. "Introduction. The Study of Mythology and Comparative Mythology." In *Myth in Indo-European Antiquity*, ed. Gerald James Larson, C. Scott Littleton and Jaan Puhvel, 1–16. Berkeley, Los Angeles, London: University of California Press, 1974.

Lebrun, François. *Se soigner autrefois. Médecins, saints, sorciers aux 17e et 18e siècles*. Paris: Temps Actuel, 1983.

Lee, D. S. "The Evening Tea Break Ritual: a Case Study" *Contemporary Nurse* 8, no. 1 (1999): 227–231.

Lehrman, Arthur. "The Miracle of St. Cosmas and St. Damian." *Plastic and Reconstructive Surgery* 94 (1994): 218–221.

Leibovici, L. "Effects of Remote, Retroactive Intercessory Prayer on Outcomes in Patients with Bloodstream Infection: Randomised Controlled Trial." *BMJ* 323, no. 7327 (2001): 1450–1451.

Lemieux, Raymond, and Micheline Milot, ed. *Les croyances des Québécois: esquisses pour une approche empirique*, Les Cahiers de recherches en sciences de la religion, no. 11. Québec: Groupe de rechereche en sciences de la religion; Les Cahiers de recherches en sciences de la religion, 1992.

Leuret, François, and Henri Bon. *Modern Miraculous Cures: A Documented Account*. Trans. John C. Barry and A. T. Macqueen. London: Peter Davies, 1957.

Lindberg, David C., and Ronald L. Numbers, ed. *When Science and Christianity Meet*. Chicago: University of Chicago Press, 2003.

Littleton, C. Scott. "Georges Dumézil and the Rebirth of the Genetic Model. An Anthropological Appreciation." In *Myth in Indo-European Antiquity*, ed. Gerald James Larson, C. Scott Littleton, and Jaan Puhvel, 169–179. Berkeley, Los Angeles, London: University of California Press, 1974.

———. *The New Comparative Mythology: An Anthropological Assessment of the Theories of Georges Dumézil*. 3rd ed. Berkeley and Los Angeles: University of California Press, 1982.

Lloyd, Geoffrey E. R. *Magic, Reason, and Experience. Studies in the Origins and Development of Greek Science*. Cambridge: Cambridge University Press, 1979.

Lloyd, Joan Barclay, and Karin Bull-Simonsen Einaudi. *SS. Cosma e Damiano in Mica Aurea: architectura, storia e storiografia di un monastero romano soppresso*. Roma: Pressa de la società alla Biblioteca Vallicelliana, 1998.

Louis, André J. *Voodoo in Haiti: Catholicism, Protestantism and a Model of Effective Ministry in the Context of Voodoo in Haiti*. Mustang, Oklahoma: Tate Publishing, 2007.

Lowe, K. J. P. *Nun's Chronicles and Convent Culture in Renaissance and Counter-Reformation Italy*. Cambridge: Cambridge University Press, 2003.

Malamut, Elizabeth. *Sur la route des saints byzantins*. Paris: CNRS, 1993.

Mangiapan, Théodore. "Le contrôle médical des guérisons à Lourdes." In *Histoire des miracles. Actes de la Sixième Rencontre d'Histoire Religieuse*, 8–9 octobre 1982, 143–164. Angers: Presses de l'Université d'Angers, 1983.

Marraffa, Giuseppe. *Santi Cosma e Damiano vita e martirio. Il Cristianismo e l'impero Romano nel II e III sec*, np, 2000.

Martellotta, Angelo. *Memorie istoriche ed il presente nel culto dei SS. Medici ricorrendo il 350° anniversario della devozione alberobellese*. Alberobello: A.G.A. Editrice, 1986.

———. *La fiera dei santi medici in Alberobello*. Fasano: Grafischena e Comitatio Feste Patronali, 1992.

Masters, Kevin S., and Glen I. Spielmans. "Prayer and Health: Review, Meta-Analysis, and Research Agenda." *Journal of Behavioral Medicine* 30, no. 4 (2007): 329–338.

Masters, Kevin S., Glen I. Spielmans, and Jason T. Goodson. "Are There Demonstrable Effects of Distant Intercessory Prayer? A Meta-Analytic Review." *Annals of Behavioral Medicine* 32, no. 1 (2006): 21–26.

Matthews, Dale A. "Religious Commitment and Health Status: A Review of the Research and Implications for Family Medicine." *Archives of Family Medicine* 7, no. Mar-Apr. (1998): 118–124.

———. "Prayer and Spirituality." *Rheumatic Diseases Clinics of North America* 26, no. February (2000): 177–187.

Matthews, D. A., S. M. Marlowe, and F. S. MacNutt. "Effects of Intercessory Prayer on Patients with Rheumatoid Arthritis." *Southern Medical Journal* 93, no. 12 (2000): 1177–1186.

Matthews, Leslie G. "SS. Cosmas and Damian—Patron Saints of Medicine and Pharmacy Their Cult in England." *Medical History* 12, no. 3 (1968): 281–288.

Meagher, Timothy J. "The Importance of Being Italian: Italian Americans in American Popular Culture, 1960s to 1990s." In *From Arrival to Incorporation: Migrants to the U.S. in a Global Era*, ed. Elliott R. Barkan, Hasia Diner, and Alan M. Kraut. New York: New York University Press, 2008.

Melinsky, Michael A. H. *Healing Miracles: An Examination from History and Experience of the Place of Miracle in Christian Thought and Medical Practice*. London: Mowbray, 1968.

Menesto, Enrico, ed. *Il processo di canonizzazione di Chiara da Montefalco*. Firenze: La Nuova Italia, 1984.

Mercado, Julian Gascon. *Breve historia del Hospital de Jesus: la más antigua institución de asistencia privada de América* 3rd ed. Mexico: Olmeca, 1985.

Miller, Timothy S. *The Birth of the Hospital in the Byzantine Empire*. Baltimore and London: Johns Hopkins University Press, 1985.

Milot, Micheline. "L'investigation du croire. Parcours et impératifs méthodologiques." In *Les Croyances des Québécois: Esquisses pour une approche*, ed. Raymond Lemieux and Micheline Milot, 93–114. Québec: Groupe de rechereche en sciences de la religion; Les Cahiers de recherches en sciences de la religion, no. 11, 1992.

Montserrat, Dominic. "Pilgrimage to the Shrine of SS Cyrus and John at Menouthis in Late Antiquity." In *Pilgrimage and Holy Space in Late Antique Egypt*, ed. David Frankfurter, 257–279. Leiden, Boston, Köln: Brill, 1998.

Mooney, Margarita A. *Faith Makes Us Live: Surviving and Thriving in the Haitian Diaspora*. Berkeley, University of California Press, 2009.

Morea, Domenico. *Il culto dei SS. MM. Cosmo e Damiano nella chiesa parrochiale di Alberobello*. Napoli: Ristampa Anastatica, [1886] 1992.

Müller, M. L'Abbé Eug. "Inventaire de la Collégiale Saint-Cosme de Luzarches aux XIVe et XVe siècles." Pontoise: Imprimerie de Amédée Paris, Lucien Paris, successeur, 1893.

Mullin, Richard. *Miracles and Magic: The Miracles and Spells of Saints and Witches*. London and Oxford: Mowbray, 1979.

Mullin, Robert Bruce. *Miracles and the Modern Religious Imagination.* New Haven and London: Yale University Press, 1996.

———. "Science, Miracles, and the Prayer Gauge Debate." In *When Science and Christianity Meet*, ed. David C. Lindberg and Ronald L. Numbers, 203–224. Chicago: University of Chicago Press, 2003.

Muriel, Josefina. *Hospitales de la Nueva España Tomo I: Fundaciones del Siglo XVI.* Mexico, 1956.

———. "Los hospitales de la Nueva España en el siglo XVI." In *Medicina novohispana. Tomo II*, ed. Gonzalo Aguirre Betrán and Roberto Moreno de los Arcos, 228–254. Mexico: Academia Nacional de Medicina y Universidad Nacional Autónoma de Mexico, 1990.

———. *Hospitales de la Nueva España Tomo II: Fundaciones de los Siglos XVII y XVIII.* Mexico: Universidad Nacional Autónoma de México and Cruz Roja Mexicana, 1991.

Numbers, Ronald L., and Darrel W. Amundsen, ed. *Caring and Curing. Health and Medicine in the Western Religious Traditions.* New York and London: Macmillan, 1986.

O'Connell, Marvin R. "The Roman Catholic Tradition since 1545." In *Caring and Curing. Health and Medicine in the Western Religious Traditions*, ed. Ronald L. Numbers and Darrel W. Amundsen, 108–145. New York and London: Macmillan, 1986.

Orsi, Robert A. *The Madonna of 115th Street: Faith and Community in Italian Harlem.* New Haven and London: Yale University Press, 1985.

———. "'He Keeps Me Going': Women's Devotion to Saint Jude Thaddeus and the Dialectics of Gender in American Catholicism, 1929–1965." In *Belief in History: Innovative Approaches to European and American Religion*, ed. Thomas Kselman, 137–169. Notre Dame and London: University of Notre Dame Press, 1991.

———. *Thank You, St. Jude: Women's Devotion to the Patron Saint of Hopeless Causes.* New Haven and London: Yale University Press, 1994.

———. "The Religious Boundaries of an In-Between People: Street *Feste* and the Problem of the Dark-Sinned Other in Italian Harlem, 1920–1990." In *Gods of the City; Religion and the American Urban Landscape*, ed. Robert A. Orsi, 257–88. Bloomington and Indianapolis: Indiana University Press, 1999.

Overall, Christine. "Miracles as Evidence against the Existence of God." *Southern Journal of Philosophy* 23, no.3 (1985): 347–53.

Park, Katharine. *Secrets of Women: Gender, Generation, and the Origins of Human Dissection.* Cambridge, Mass.: Zone Books and MIT Press, 2006.

Park, R. H. R. and M. P. Park. "Saint Vitus' Dance: Vital Misconceptions by Sydenham and Bruegel." *Journal of the Royal Society of Medicine* 83, no. 8 (1990): 512–515.

Pazzano, Cosimo, and Domenico Capponi. *I Santi Medici Cosimo e Damiano. Vita e miracoli. Storia, culto, e religosità poplare del santuario di Riace.* Reggio di Calabria: Laruffa Editore, 2000.

Peck, Edward, Perri Six, Pauline Gulliver, and David Towell. "Why Do We Keep on Meeting Like This? The Board as Ritual in Health and Social Care." *Health Services Management Research* 17, no. 2 (2004): 100–109.

Pecker, André, ed. *La médecine à Paris du XIIIe au XXe siècle*. Paris: Editions Hervas, 1984.

Perrot, Jean. *Mythe et littérature sous le signe des jumeaux*. Paris: Presses Universitaires de la France, 1976.

Perry, M. C. "Believing the Miracles and Preaching the Resurrection [1962]." In *The Miracles and the Resurrection; Some Recent Studies*, ed. Ian T. Ramsey, G. H. Boobyer, F. N. Davey, M. C. Perry and Henry Cadbury, J., 31–49. London: S.P.C.K.; Theological Collections no. 3, 1964.

Peschel, Richard E., and Enid Rhodes Peschel. "Medical Miracles from a Physician-Scientist's Viewpoint." *Perspectives in Biology and Medicine* 31, no. 3 (1988): 391–404.

Philpin, Susan. "'Handing Over': Transmission of Information between Nurses in an Intensive Therapy Unit." *Nursing in Critical Care* 11, no. 2 (2006): 86–93.

Philippi, Donald L. *Kojiki*. Tokyo: Tokyo University Press, 1968.

Pick, Bernard. *The Apocryphal Acts of Paul, Peter, John, Andrew and Thomas*. Chicago: Open Court Publishing, 1909.

Pickstone, J. V. "Establishment and Dissent in Nineteenth-Century Medicine: An Exploration of Some Correspondence and Connections between Religious and Medical Belief Systems." In *The Church and Healing*, ed. W. J. Sheils, 165–189. Oxford: Basil Blackwell and The Ecclesiastical History Society, 1982.

Preston, James J. "Necessary Fictions: Healing Encounters with a North American Saint." *Literature and Medicine* 8 (1989): 42–62.

Procopius. *Buildings*. Trans. H. B. Dewing. 7 vols. Vol. 7. Cambridge, Mass.: Harvard University Press. Loeb Classical Library, 1914.

Puchalski, C. M., and D. B. Larson. "Developing Curricula in Spirituality and Medicine." *Academic Medicine* 73, no. 9 (1998): 970–974.

Ramsey, Ian T. "Miracles: An Exercise in Logical Mapwork [1952]." In *The Miracles and the Resurrection: Some Recent Studies*, ed. Ian T. Ramsey, G. H. Boobyer, F. N. Davey, M. C. Perry, and Henry J. Cadbury, 1–30. London: S.P.C.K.; Theological Collections no. 3, 1964.

Remus, Harold. *Pagan Christian conflict over Miracle in the Second Century*. Cambridge, Mass.: The Philadelphia Patristic Foundation, 1983.

Renouard, Michel, and Nathalie Merrien. *Saints guérisseurs de Bretagne*. Rennes: Editions-Ouest France, 1994.

Renzi, Salvatore de. *Storia documentata della scuola medica di Salerno*. 2nd ed. Naples: Gaetano Nobile, 1857.

Resch, Andreas. *Miracoli dei Beati, 1983–1990*. Città del Vaticano: Libreria Editrice Vaticano, 2002.

———. *Miracoli dei Beati, 1991–1995*. Città del Vaticano: Libreria Editrice Vaticano, 2002.

———. *Miracoli dei Santi, 1983–1995*. Città del Vaticano: Libreria Editrice Vaticano, 2002.

Rey, Terry. "Toward an Ethnohistory of Haitian Pilgrimage." *Journal de la Société des Américainistes* 9, no. 1 (2005): 161–183.

———. "Catholic Pentecostalism in Haiti: Spirit, Politics, and Gender." *Pneuma* 32, no. 1 (2010): 80–106.

Riis, Ole Preben. "Methodology in the Sociology of Religion." In *The Oxford Handbook of the Sociology of Religion*, ed. Peter B. Clarke, 229–243. Oxford: Oxford University Press, 2009.

Risse, Guenter B. *Mending Bodies, Saving Souls: A History of Hospitals*. New York and Oxford: Oxford University Press, 1999.

Roberts, L., I. Ahmed, and S. Hall. "Intercessory Prayer for the Alleviation of Ill Health." *Cochrane Database of Systematic Reviews* 2, no. CD000368 (2000).

———. "Intercessory Prayer for the Alleviation of Ill Health." *Cochrane Database of Systematic Reviews* 1, no. CD000368 (2007).

Roberts, Leanne, Irshad Ahmed, Steve Hall, and Andrew. Davison. "Intercessory Prayer for the Alleviation of Ill Health." *Cochrane Database of Systematic Reviews* 2, no. CD000368 (2009).

Rodriguez, Martha Eugenia. "Un espacio para la atención del indígena. El hospital real de naturales." In *Pensiamento novohispano 7*, ed. Noé Esquivel Estrada, 105–116. Toluca, Mexico: Universidad Autónoma del Estado de México, 2006.

Romanoff, Bronna D., and Barbara E. Thompson. "Meaning Construction in Palliative Care: the Use of Narrative, Ritual, and the Expressive Arts" *American Journal of Hospice & Palliative Medicine* 23, no. 4 (2006): 309–316.

Rossi, Francesco, Mario Mangrella, Anna Loffreda, and Enrico Lampa. "Wizards and Scientists: The Pharmacologic Experience in the Middle Ages." *American Journal of Nephrology* 14 (1994): 384–390.

Roush, Wade. "Herbert Benson: Mind-Body Maverick Pushes the Envelope." 1997 *Science* 276 no. 5311 (1997): 357.

Rousselle, Robert. "Healing Cults in Antiquity: The Dream Cures of Asclepius of Epidaurus." *Journal of Psychohistory* 12, no. Winter 1985 (1984–5): 339–352.

Running, Alice, Lauren W. Tolle, and Deb Girard. "Ritual: the Final Expression of Care." *International Journal of Nursing Practice* 14, no. 4 (2008): 303–307.

Rupprecht, Ernest. *Cosmae et Damiani sanctorum medicorum vitam et miracula e codice Londinensi*. Berlin: Junker und Dünnhaupt Verlag, 1935.

Russo, Francesco. *Regesto Vaticano per la Calabria*. 10 vols. Roma: Gesuladi Editore, 1974–1986.

Sabourin, Leopold. *The Divine Miracles Discussed and Defended*. Rome: Catholic Book Agency, 1977.

Salleron, Louis. "Le miracle. Des évangiles à Lourdes." In *Histoire des miracles. Actes de la Sixième Rencontre d'Histoire Religieuse*, 8–9 octobre 1982, ed. Centre de recherches d'histoire religieuse et d'histoire des idées Université d'Angers, 179–191. Angers: Presses de l'Université d'Angers, 1983.

Schlich, Thomas. "How Gods and Saints Became Transplant Surgeons: The Scientific Article as a Model for the Writing of History." *History of Science* xxxiii (1995): 311–331.

Schwartz, Hillel. *The Culture of the Copy: Striking Likenesses, Unreasonable Facsimiles.* New York: Zone Books, 1996.

Schwartz, Richard S., F. Roy Mackintosh, Jerry Halpern, Stanley L. Schrier, and Peter L. Greenberg. "Multivariate Analysis of Factors Associated with Outcome of Treatment for Adults with Acute Myelogenous Leukemia." *Cancer* 54 (1984): 1672–1681.

Sciorra, Joseph. ""We Go Where the Italians Live": Religious Processions as Ethnic and Territorial Markers in a Multi-Ethnic Brooklyn Neighborhood." In *Gods of the City; Religion and the American Urban Landscape*, ed. Robert A. Orsi, 310–340. Bloomington and Indianapolis: Indiana University Press, 1999.

Scott, Robert A. *Miracle Cures: Saints Pilgrimage and the Healing Powers of Belief.* Berkeley: University of California Press, 2010.

Shaw, Jane. *Miracles in Enlightenment England.* New Haven, CT: Yale University Press, 2006.

Shahid, Irfan. "Arab-Christian Pilgrimages in the Proto-Byzantine Period (V-VII Centuries)." In *Pilgrimage and Holy Space in Late Antique Egypt*, ed. David Frankfurter, 373–389. Leiden, Boston, Köln: Brill, 1998.

Shoemaker, Innis Howe. "An Interview with William H. Helfand." In *Health for Sale: Posters from the William H. Helfand Collection*, 7–16. Philadelphia: Philadelphia Museum of Art, 2011.

Sicher, Fred, Elisabeth Targ, Dan Moore II, and Helene S. Smith. "A Randomized Double-Blind Study of the Effect of Distant Healing in a Population with Advanced AIDS. Report of a Small-Scale Study." *Western Journal of Medicine* 169 (1998): 356–363.

Sigal, Pierre André. *L'homme et le miracle dans la France médievale.* Paris: Editions du Cerf, 1985.

Simons, Marlise. "Spiritual Values. Why Catholics are Flocking to Shrines." *Globe and Mail*, October 14, 1993, A21.

Skinner, Patricia. *Health and Medicine in Early Medieval Southern Italy.* Leiden, New York, Köln: Brill, 1996.

Skrobucha, Heinz. *The Patrons of the Doctors.* Trans. Hans Hermann Rosenwald, Pictoral Library of Eastern Church Art, vol. 7. Recklinghausen, West Germany: Aurel Bongers, 1965.

Sloan, R. P., E. Bagiella, and T. Powell. "Religion, Spirituality, and Medicine." *Lancet* 353, no. February 20 (1999): 664–667.

Sloan, Richard P., and Rajasekhar Ramakrishnan. "Science, Medicine, and Intercessory Prayer." *Perspectives in Biology & Medicine* 49, no. 4 (2006): 504–514.

Somolinos d'Ardois, Germán. "Médicos y libros en el primer siglo de la Colonia." In *Medicina novohispana. Tomo II*, ed. Gonzalo Aguirre Betrán and Roberto Moreno de los Arcos, 159–174. Mexico: Academia Nacional de Medicina y Universidad Nacional Autónoma de Mexico, 1990.

Sonnenberg, A. "Personal View: Cost and Benefit of Medical Rituals in Gastroenterology." *Alimentary Pharmacology & Therapeutics* 20, no. 9 (2004): 939–942.

Sournia, Jean-Charles, and Marianne Sournia. *L'orient des premiers chrétiens: histoire et archéologie de la Syrie byzantine.* Paris: Fayard, 1966.

Souverbie, M. T. "Magie et médecine." *Histoire de la Médecine,* 20 mars 1970, 3–43.

Stanger-Ross, Jordan. *Staying Italian: Urban Change and Ethnic Life in Postwar Toronto and Philadelphia.* Chicago and London: University of Chicago Press, 2009.

Stiltingo, Joanne. "De SS Cosma, Damiano, Anthimo, Leontio et Euprepio MM. Aegis in Cilicia." In *Acta Sanctorum Septembris,* 428–478. Antwerp: Bernardum Alb. Vander Plassche, 1760.

Sudhoff, Karl. "Healing Miracles of SS. Cosmas-Damian and Cyrus-John." In *Essays in the History of Medicine,* ed. Fielding H. Garrison, 219–221. New York: Medical Life Press, 1926.

Sulmasy, Daniel P. "What Is a Miracle?" *Southern Medical Journal* 100, no. 12 (2007): 1223–1228.

Swinburne, Richard. *The Concept of Miracle.* London and Basingstoke: Macmillan St. Martin's, 1970.

Szabo, Jason. "Seeing Is Believing? The Form and Substance of French Medical Debates over Lourdes." *Bulletin of the History of Medicine* 76 (2002): 199–230.

Tacitus. "Germania." In *Tacitus in Five Volumes,* ed. M. Hutton and E. H. Warmington, vol. 1. Cambridge, Mass. and London: Harvard University Press and Heinemann, 1980.

Taviani-Carozzi, Huguette. *La principauté lombarde de Salerne (IXe-XIe siècle): pouvoir et société en Italie lombarde méridionale.* 2 vols. Rome and Paris: Ecole française de Rome and De Boccard, 1991.

Tejirian, Edward J. *Sexuality and the Devil.* New York and London: Routledge, 1990.

Temkin, Owsei, *Hippocrates in a World of Pagans and Christians.* Baltimore: Johns Hopkins University Press, 1991.

Temperini, Lino. *Basilica Santi Cosma e Damiano Roma.* Trans. Seraphin Conley. Rome: Franciscanum Casa Generalizia TOR and MC grafica, nd [ca. 1995].

———. *Santi Cosma e Damiano medici martiri.* Roma: Editrice Franciscanum, 1997.

Theodoret de Cyr. *Thérapeutique des maladies helléniques.* Trans. Pierre Canivet. 2 vols. Paris: Cerf, 1958.

Théodoridès, Jean. "Saints in Medical History (a complement)." *Clio Medica* 14 (1979): 269–270.

Thomas, Keith Vivian. *Religion and the Decline of Magic.* New York: Charles Scribner's Sons, 1971.

Thurston, Herbert, and Donald Attwater. "Cosmas and Damian." In *Butler's Lives of the Saints,* 659–660. New York: P. J. Kenedy & Sons, 1963.

Travlos, John. *Pictorial Dictionary of Ancient Athens.* London: Thames and Hudson, 1971.

Trenard, Louis. "Les miracles ralliés par Voltaire." In *Histoire des miracles. Actes de la Sixième Rencontre d'Histoire Religieuse, 8–9 octobre 1982,* ed. Centre de recherches d'histoire religieuse et d'histoire des idées Université d'Angers, 95–109. Angers: Presses de l'Université d'Angers, 1983.

Tripputi, Anna Maria. *Bibliografia degli ex voto*. Bari: Paolo Malagrino, 1995.

Tucci, Pier Luigi. "The Revival of Antiquity in Medieval Rome: The Restoration of the Basilica of Cosmas and Damian in the Twelfth Century." *Memoirs of the American Academy in Rome* 49 (2004): 99–126.

———. "Eight Fragments of the Marble Plan of Rome Shedding New Light on the Transtiberim." *Papers of the British School at Rome* 72 (2004): 185–202.

Turner, D. D. "Just Another Drug? A Philosophical Assessment of Randomised Controlled Studies on Intercessory Prayer." *Journal of Medical Ethics* 32, no. 8 (2006): 487–490.

United States. Armed Forces Medical Library. *Subject Heading Authority List*. Washington, DC: U.S. Government Printing Office, 1954.

Université d'Angers, Centre de recherches d'histoire religieuse et d'histoire des idées, ed. *Histoire des miracles. Actes de la Sixième Rencontre d'Histoire Religieuse, 8–9 octobre 1982*. Angers: Presses de l'Université d'Angers, 1983.

Vacca, Domenico. *Reading the Life of the Holy Doctors: Cosma and Damiano*. Trans. Joseph DeCandia. Bitonto, 1973.

Van Dam, Raymond. *Saints and their Miracles in Late Antique Gaul*. Princeton, N.J.: Princeton University Press, 1993.

Varacalli, Joseph A., Salvatore Primeggia, Salvatore LaGumina, and Donald J. D'Elia, ed. *The Saints in the Lives of Italian-Americans: An Interdisciplinary Investigation*, Filibrary No. 14. Stony Brook, N.Y.: Forum Italicum, Supplement, 1999.

Vauchez, André. *La sainteté en occident aux derniers siècles du Moyen Age d'après les proces de canonisation et les documents hagiographiques*. Rome: Ecole française de Rome, 1981.

Veith, Ilza. "Twin Birth: Blessing or Disaster. A Japanese View." *International Journal of Social Psychiatry* 6 (1960): 230–236.

Viguerie, Jean de. "Les caractères permanents du miracle." In *Histoire des miracles. Actes de la Sixième Rencontre d'Histoire Religieuse, 8–9 octobre 1982*, ed. Jean de Viguerie, 193–200. Angers: Presses de l'Université d'Angers, 1983.

Vilarrasa i Coch, Josep M. *Els Sants Metges guaridors, Sant Cosme i Sant Damià: història, llegenda i goigs*. Barcelona: Editorial Mediterrània, 2004.

Voragine, Jacobus de. "Cosmas and Damian." In *The Golden Legend*, 575–578. New York, London, Toronto: Longmans, Green and Co., 1969.

Wall, B. M. "Science and Ritual: the Hospital as Medical and Sacred Space, 1865–1920." *Nursing History Review* 11 (2003): 51–68.

Wallis, Faith. "The Experience of the Book: Manuscripts, Texts, and the Role of Epistemology in Early Medieval Medicine." In *Knowledge and the Scholarly Medical Traditions*, ed. Don Bates, 101–126. Cambridge: Cambridge University Press, 1995.

Ward, Donald. *The Divine Twins. An Indo-European Myth in Germanic Tradition*. Berkeley and Los Angeles: University of California Press, 1968.

———. "The Separate Functions of the Indo-European Divine Twins." In *Myth and Law among the Indo-Europeans*, ed. Jaan Puhvel, 193–202. Berkeley, London, Los Angeles: University of California Press, 1970.

Wasserug, Joseph D. "It's a Miracle!" *Postgraduate Medicine* 86, no. 1 (1989): 76–77.

Webster, Charles. "Paracelsus Confronts the Saints: Miracles, Healing, and the Secularization of Magic." *Social History of Medicine* 7, no. 3 (1995): 403–421.

Wedel, Johan. *Santería Healing: A Journey into the Afro-Cuban World of Divinities, Spirits, and Sorcery*. Gainesville: University Press of Florida, 2004.

Whittaker, J. A., P. Reizenstein, Sheila T. Callender, G. G. Cornwell, I. W. Delamore, R. P. Gale, M. Gobbi, P. Jacobs, B. Lantz, A. T. Maiolo, J. K. H. Rees, E. J. Van Slyck, and H. Vu Van. "Long Survival in Acute Myelogenous Leukaemia: an Internal Collaborative Study." *British Medical Journal* 282, no. 6265 (1981): 692–695.

Williams, T. C. *The Idea of the Miraculous: The Challenge to Science and Religion*. Basingstoke and London: Macmillan, 1990.

Wilstach, Paul. "The Stone Beehive Homes of the Italian Heel: in Trulli-Land the Native Builds His Dwelling and Makes his Field Arable in the Same Operation." *National Geographic* 57, no. 2 (1930): 228–260.

Wittmann, Anneliese. *Kosmas und Damian. Kultausbreitung und Volksdevotion*. Berlin: E. Schmidt, 1967.

Woodward, Kenneth L. *Making Saints. How the Catholic Church Determines Who Becomes a Saint and Who Doesn't, and Why*. New York: Simon and Schuster, 1990.

———. *The Book of Miracles; The Meaning of the Miracle Stories in Christianity, Judaism, Buddhism, Hinduism, Islam*. New York: Simon and Schuster, 2000.

York, Glyn Y. "Religious-Based Denial in the NICU: Implications for Social Work." *Social Work in Health Care* 12, no. 4 (1987): 31–45.

Zimmerman, Kees W., ed. *One Leg in the Grave; The Miracle of the Transplantation of the Black Leg*. Maarsen: Elsevier/Bunge, 1998.

Zucchi, John E. *Italians in Toronto: Development of a National Identity, 1875–1935*. Montreal and Kingston: McGill Queen's University Press, 1988.

Zuring, J. *De heilige genezers Cosmas en Damianus in Nederland*. Venlo: Van Spijk, 1989.

Index

Acta Sanctorum, 33, 34, 39
Acts of Thomas, 45
Africa, 40, 52, 150, 152, 153, 158, 162, 172
Agatha, St, 132
Agrigento, Sicily, 103, 104, 106
AIDS, 120
Alberobello, Italy, 54, 55, 56, 71, 86, 98,
    111–17, 119, 135, 172, 184
Alci, twins, 44
Aleppo, 36
Alexandria, 44
Allard, Pierre-Paul, 12, 13
Amalfi Coast, 121–26
American Association for the History of
    Medicine, 93, 155, 158
American Medical Association, 56
American Osler Society, 155, 159, 160
Amerindians, 52, 92, 152, 172
Amsterdam, 61, 62
Anagni, Italy, 123
Anargyroi, 33, 37, 167
Andes, Stephen, 134
Andrew, St., 125
Angela Merici, St., 130
Annese photographers, 115
Anthony of Padua, St., 21, 54
    See also churches
archeology, 24, 34, 103, 160

Argentina, 40
artists, 42, 100, 108, 147
Asia, 40
Asklepios, 36, 43, 45, 98, 103, 104, 122
Assisi, Italy, 20, 22, 23
Asvins (Nasatyas) twins, 44
atheists, 100, 140, 145, 160, 169, 176–77
Athens, 38
Atulino, Bartholomew, 107
Auer rod, 3, 5
Australia, 145, 162
Austria, 40

Barcelona, Spain, 99, 156
Barí, Italy, 75, 76, 83, 86, 119, 120, 184
basilicas to Sts. Cosmas and Damian
    Rome, 24, 38–39, 40, 41, 42, 43, 133,
      135, 158, 160–62
    Bitonto, 119
    Alberobello, 112
    See also churches; St. Peter's Basilica
Bastide, Roger, 152
Beaulieu, Thérèse, 70
Belgium, 33, 168
Bellegarde-Smith, Patrick, 150
Benedict XVI, Pope, 9, 16
Benedict, St., 38
Bennett, Gillian, 62

Benson, Herbert, 143
Bessette, Alfred. *See* Frère André
Billingsley, Ian, 79
Bitonto, 86, 111, 117–21, 135, 173
black leg, miracle of, 37, 38, 124, 128, 161
Boer, Witse de, 62
Botticelli, Sandro, 42
Bouchaud, Constantin, priest, 23, 26, 27, 130, 131
Bourget, Monsignor Ignace, 70
Brazil, 40, 41, 152, 153, 161
Bremen, Germany, 39
Brittany, France, 100
Bronx, N.Y., 86, 88
Brooklyn, N.Y., 148–49
Brown, Elizabeth A. (Peggy), 134
Brown, Peter R. L., 45
Bulgaria, 40
Byzantine traditions, 37, 40, 73, 103, 104, 110, 111

caduceus, 56
Calabria, 71, 83, 84, 86, 110
Cambridge, Mass., 80–83, 84, 86, 88, 95, 102, 103, 135, 149
Canadian Ambassador to Holy See, 23, 25, 162
Canadian Society for the History of Medicine, 52–54
cancer, 87, 88, 120, 163, 180–84
Cannito, Giuseppe, 117
canonization, 9, 11, 12, 18, 19, 25, 63, 95, 162–63, 175–76
    ceremony of, 26
    miracles in, 129–33, 135
    rules of, 9, 29
Carrel, Alexis, 158
Carroll, Michael P., 84
Casey, Sister Mary, 162
Castor and Pollux (Dioscuri), 24, 43, 45, 51, 53, 98, 104, 111, 133, 135, 163
    myth of, 43–44

Catalonia, 99, 155, 156
Cataudella, Julia, 79, 82–83, 88, 102, 137, 138, 145, 148–49
Celts, 100, 111
charity, 76, 82, 98, 120
Charlottetown, P.E.I., 53, 58
Christianity, early, 24, 36–39, 44, 45–46, 53, 152, 167, 170
churches
    of the Most Precious Blood, Manhattan, 71–73
    of Our Lady of Grace Church, Howard Beach, N.Y., 74–75
    of St. Anthony of Padua, Utica, N.Y., 54
    of St. Francis, Toronto, 31, 32, 33, 46, 47–51, 67, 71, 172
    of Sts. Cosmas and Damian, Conshohocken, 147–48
    of Sts. Cosmas and Damian, Eboli, 126
    of Sts. Cosmas and Damian, Isernia, 128
    of Sts. Cosmas and Damian, Mexico, 91, 92
    of Sts. Cosmas and Damian, Riace, 107–9
    of Sts. Cosmas and Damian, Rome, 40, 133
    of Sts. Cosmas and Damian, San Cosmo Albanese, 110–11
    See also basilicas
Citò, Giorgio, 115
Clara of the Cross, St., 131, 132
Clara, St., 22
clinical trials, 142–45, 165, 166, 171
Cochrane Systemic Reviews, 144
Collège Saint Côme, 41
conferences, 52–54, 61–63, 90, 93, 94, 120, 143, 155, 158, 160, 161
confraternities, 98, 100, 107, 108, 109, 112, 113, 114, 116
Confrérie Saint Cosme, 100

Conshohocken, PA, 147–50, 153
Constantine the African, 123
Constantine, Roman Emperor 36
Constantinople, 37, 104, 135
Cordoba, Spain, 40
Cortes, Hernando, 92
Cosmas and Damian, Sts. and doctors, 21, 24
  in Cambridge, 80–83
  in Conshohocken, 147–50
  as doctors, 21, 30, 31, 51, 52, 53, 70, 71, 79, 84–86, 89, 94, 95, 116, 136, 154
  feast day of, 43
  historical veneration of, 36–43
  in Howard Beach, 73–79
  in Italy, 101–29
  lives of, 33–34
  in Manhattan, 71–73
  as Marassa, 150–53
  martyrdom of, 34, 35, 85, 163
  in Mexico, 89–92
  miracles of, 37, 42, 44, 62, 69, 76, 80, 86–89, 120, 121, 128, 181–84
  mosaic of, 24, 39, 41
  "oldest" shrine of, 107, 117, 124, 133, 135
  in Québec, 69–71
  relics of, 39, 40, 80, 98, 100, 104, 107, 109, 111, 112, 114, 116, 119–20, 125, 135, 158
  role of, 135, 172–73
  Roman basilica of, 24, 38–39, 40, 41, 42, 43, 133, 135, 158, 160–62
  societies for, 71, 72, 73, 75–77, 79, 80, 81, 98, 100, 107–9, 112–14, 116, 121, 128
  and theories, 51–52, 53, 58, 59, 65, 95, 121, 135–36, 172–73
  in Toronto, 31–33, 46–51, 53, 62, 66–68, 69, 79–80, 83, 84, 86, 93–94, 172–73
  as twins, 84–85, 154, 179
  in Utica, 54–57

  in Vatican Archives, 132
  See also churches; healing; miracles; statues
Croatia, 40
Cyprian, St. and doctor, 167
Cyrrhus (Cyr), 34, 36, 37
Cyrus and John, Sts. and doctors, 44
Czech Republic, 40

David-Danel, Marie-Louise, 42, 98, 100
death, 51–52, 133, 140, 154, 163, 166–67, 170
DeCandia, Joe and Clara, 76–79, 155, 173
degradation narrative, 45
Delehaye, Hippolyte, 45
demons, 131, 132
Denmark, 144
DeNonno, Tony, 146
Devil's Advocate, 9, 17
diagnosis, 3, 5, 6, 7, 9, 10, 13, 14, 52, 87, 132, 171
DiDomenico, Sal, 81
diffusion, 53, 58, 84, 95, 135
Diocletion, Roman Emperor, 33, 34, 36
Dioscuri. *See* Castor and Pollux
Dioscurism, universal, 51, 154
Dischiavo, William, Deacon, 54–57, 58, 59, 68, 71, 112
diseases, 37, 87–88, 120, 130–31, 132–33
  as ideas, 29, 140, 171
Drotbohm, Heike, 150, 151
Drouin, Jeanne, 5, 7–11, 14, 18, 19, 23, 25, 26, 27
Durkheim, Emile, 52, 63

Eboli, 122, 126–27
Egypt, 40, 52
Elder, Rachel, 149
epidemics, 40, 99, 106, 112, 135
epilepsy, 125, 130, 167
ethics, 65, 120, 145, 166
Evans, Francis J., priest, 75, 76, 155

evidence
  historical, 9, 25, 33, 44, 45, 46, 53, 95,
    104
  and miracles, 21, 26, 50, 142, 166, 169
  scientific, 7, 10, 64, 136, 171

feast-day celebrations, 65, 66, 99, 153,
    179–80
  in Canada, 47–48, 53–54, 86, 172
  in Italy, 103, 104, 107–9, 112–17, 119,
    126, 128, 129
  in the United States, 55, 58, 59, 71, 72,
    77, 81, 86, 146–50
Feldberg, Gina, 58, 61
Felix IV, Pope, 38
Ferland-Angers, Albertine, 15
Festugière, André Jean, 45
Filippo Benizi, St. and doctor, 133
Florence, 20, 21, 42, 126
Fra Angelico, 35, 42, 124
France, 65, 97–100
Francis of Assisi, St., 22–23, 71, 111
  See also churches
Franklin, Benjamin, 168
Frère André, St., 17, 162, 163, 175
Freud, Sigmund, 119
Fromicini, Orsola, 40
Fye, Bruce, 158

Gabriel of the Sorrowful Virgin, St., 130
Gaeta, Italy, 81, 82, 86, 87, 98, 101, 102–3,
    135
Galen, 123, 160, 161
Gallouin, François and Martine, 99
Gardy, Albert, priest, 149
gender, 83, 94, 114, 123
genealogical theory, 51, 53, 54, 95, 107,
    135, 154
Geneva, 101, 130
Gennaro (Januarius), St., 72, 125
George, St., 71
Germain, St., 40

Germany, 40, 42, 44
Gianna Beretta Molla, St. and doctor, 133
giglio, feast of, 146–47
Gijswijt-Hofstra, Marijke, 62
Girona, 99
Goering, Joseph, 94
goigs, 99, 155, 156
Golden Legend, 34
Goupil, René, St. and doctor, 26
Greece, influence of, 33, 103, 110, 122, 126
  See also Magna Graecia
Greek, manuscripts in, 37, 42, 123
Gregory the Great, Pope, 39, 161
Grey Nuns (Sisters of Charity of
    Montreal), 7–12, 15–17, 19, 25, 26, 28
  name of, 16
Grmek, Mirko, 4, 26, 89
Gruttaroti, Damiano and Beatrice,
    128–29
Guardiani, Francesco, 94
Guiscard, Robert, 122

Hagia Sofia, 38
Haïti, 25, 83, 95, 148–54, 162, 163, 172
Hamilton, William, 128
Hansen, Bert, 74, 80, 146, 148, 155, 157
healing, 61, 89
  masses for, 55, 82, 91
  physical, 46, 57, 69, 87, 89, 92, 120, 121,
    124, 171
  spiritual, 57, 69, 82, 125
  See also miracles
heart disease, 76, 80, 87, 117, 120, 143
Helfand, William, 155, 156
hematology, 3, 4, 7, 9, 14, 23, 29, 129
heroes, 13, 36, 43–44
Hinduism, 44, 141
Hippocrates, 123, 137, 167, 170
hospitals, 37, 90, 92, 120, 122, 128, 133,
    155, 157
Howard Beach, N.Y., 73–79, 82, 83, 84,
    86, 121, 135, 155

Huisman, Frank, 63
Hurbon, Laennec, 152

Iacovetta, Franca, 58, 59, 61, 68, 79, 138
Ibeji (Ibeye), twins, 150, 153
immigrants, 50, 51, 52, 54, 55, 65, 81, 94,
    122, 128, 129, 147, 172
incorruptibility of corpses, 131
incubation, 36–37, 38, 53, 88, 89, 161
India, 44
Indo-European culture, 44, 51, 52
interviews, 49–51, 58, 67, 68, 75, 80
    See also surveys
Isernia, 50, 53, 98, 127–8, 135, 172
Isis, 44, 52
Italy
    travel in, 20–22, 97, 101–29, 158–63
    See also pilgrims, origins of; *and by*
    place name

Jannetta, Ersilia, 50–51, 127, 155, 173
Japan, 52, 172
Jerusalem, 36, 38
Jesuit Martyrs, Sts., 26, 47
Jesus, 36, 39, 43, 45–46, 147
Jesus Hospital, Mexico, 92
Jews, 11, 17, 26, 37, 58, 85, 122
Joan of Arc, St., 130
John Chrysostom, St., 44, 73
John Paul II, Pope, 17, 26, 27, 28, 130, 177
Johnston, Anita, 46, 47, 49–50, 129
Joseph Moscati, St. and doctor, 133
Julian the Apostate, Roman Emperor, 36
Julien, Pierre, 42–43, 51, 98–99, 101, 102,
    111, 115, 155
Justinian, Roman Emperor, 37, 104
Juturna Fountain, 24, 43, 53, 133, 160

Kosmidion, 37

Laennec, René, 100
Lambertini, Prospero. *See* Benedict XIV

Leahy, Anne, 162
Leccese, Anthony, 80
Lella, Joseph, 54
Letourneau, Marguerite, 19, 25, 28–29
leukemia, 3, 10, 29, 131
    diagnosis of, 5–6, 7
    survival in, 6, 10, 12, 13, 14
Levi, Carlo, 126
Lippi, Filippo, 42
Lipton-Duffin, Joshua, 58
Lombardi, Giulia, 161
Lopez, Pedro, 92
Louis XIII, King, 41
Lucy, St., 132
Luke, St., and doctor, 24, 119, 125
Luzarches, France, 39, 99–100

Mackillop, Mary, St., 162, 163, 175
Madrid, 39
magic, 45, 61, 62–64, 167, 169–70
Magna Graecia, 51, 73, 103, 104, 111, 122
Maloney, Gilles, 54
Manhattan, N.Y., 59, 71–73, 83, 85, 86,
    110, 111, 148, 155
Marassa, twins, 150–53, 160
Marena, Aurelio, 119
Marguerite de Bourgeoys, St., 26
Marie-Marguerite d'Youville, St., 8, 9, 11,
    14, 17, 18, 22, 23, 25, 26, 28, 74, 129,
    162, 169, 175
    life of, 15–16
Marland, Hilary, 63
Martellotta, Angelo, 112, 127
Martellotta, Giovanni, priest, 116
martyrs, 34, 39, 42, 44
Matthews, Dale A., 143
Mayo Clinic, 155–58, 161–62
McBride, Brother Mark, 158, 160–63, 170
McGill University, 70
media, 175–76
Medical Subject Headings (MeSH), 141
medicalization, 173

Medici family, 21, 42, 111, 120
medicine, 13, 16, 75–76, 79, 82, 87, 89,
	120, 131–32, 133, 137–38, 158, 162,
	163, 165–73
	errors in, 170–71
	and religion, 30, 37, 62, 63–64, 92,
		165–72
	as religion, 158
medievalists, 74, 93, 134
MEDLINE, 137–45, 167
Messina, Sicily, 103, 106
Mexico, 40, 89–92, 152
Michelangelo Buonarotti, 44, 119
Minisci, George, 71, 85
miracles, 20, 37, 57, 61, 62, 63, 76, 80,
	85–89, 94–95, 109, 120, 121, 166–68,
	180–84
	book on, 135, 166
	in canonization, 9, 29–30, 129–35,
		162–63
	criticism of, 139–40, 165, 169,
		175–76
	definitions of, 9, 29, 63, 94, 165, 169,
		176
	as healings, 129–35, 170–72, 175,
		180–84
	in medical publishing, 138–40, 141
	and science, 9, 11, 29, 129, 136, 163, 175
Moïse, Mary, 149
Monreale, Sicily, 104, 122
Monte Cassino, Italy, 101, 123
Montreal, 70, 149, 150–51, 175
	See also Grey Nuns
Mooney, Margarita, 153
Morin, Monsignor Roger, 12, 16, 19
Moulin, Anne-Marie, 90, 91
music, 47, 57, 68, 76, 77, 80, 82, 90, 94,
	113, 114, 115, 128, 155
mythology, 51–52, 172

Naples, 71, 72, 103, 107, 121–22, 123, 125
Naro, Sicily, 105–6

National Geographic, 112, 115
National Library of Medicine, 138
New York City, N.Y., 54, 153–54
	See also Manhattan
Normand, Lise (L.N.), 6–9, 11, 12, 13, 14,
	16, 23, 25, 26, 27, 29, 177
	miracle healing of, 7, 18, 131, 177
Norse tradition, 44–45
nurses, 46, 52, 64, 92, 120, 143, 149,
	162
	See also Grey Nuns

Ojeda, Christobal, 92
Oratoire St. Joseph, Montreal, 17, 47,
	175
Orestes, St. and doctor, 167
Orsi, Robert, 149
Osler, William, 158–59, 161
Ostia Antica, 19
Ottawa, 4, 5, 12, 23, 131
Overell, Anne, 134
Oxford University Press, 135

Padua, 21
pagan religion, 24, 43–44, 45, 46, 53, 152,
	154, 167, 170
Pantaleon, St., and doctor, 125
Paolino, St., 146
Paonessa, Ralph, priest, 47, 48, 57
Paraguay, 40
paralysis, 33, 37, 130
Paré, Ambroise, 168
Paris, 4, 39, 89, 98–100
Paul VI, Pope, 17, 119
Pedraza, Diego de, 92
Perdiguero, Enrique, 63
Persico, Natale, 121
Peter, St., 111
pharmacy, 21, 40, 41, 42, 90, 100, 113, 161
physicians, 4, 6–10, 40, 52, 63, 73, 80,
	92, 100, 105, 113, 142–43, 165, 169,
	170

in miracle stories, 87, 88, 89, 131–32
in Rome (Consulta Medica), 10, 13, 14, 175
as saints, 125, 132–33, 185–87
in Salerno, 122, 123
as witnesses, 11, 15, 27, 132, 171
pilgrimage, 22, 34, 57, 69, 89, 149, 153–54, 155, 171, 172
pilgrims, 36, 64, 140, 165, 166
in Canada, 48, 67–68, 70, 137, 149
in Europe, 21, 108, 113, 119, 120, 124, 160
for health, 125–26, 173
origins of, 83, 84, 148, 149, 179
surveys of, 61–95
in the United States, 56, 57, 58, 59, 71–83, 148, 149, 153
Pio of Pietrelcina (Padre Pio), St., 79, 113, 139
Pius IX, Pope, 103
placebo, 64, 142
plague, 99, 106, 112
Poland, 26, 40, 84
polio, 55, 57
Pollack, Ann, 101
Ponce, Alonso, priest, 92
Portugal, 40
Positio super miraculo, 23, 130, 131
positivism, 64, 142, 154, 169
Potter, Paul, 54
Prague, 40
prayer, 14, 27, 38, 55, 57, 76, 79, 84, 87, 109, 114, 137, 141–42, 153–54, 160–61, 166–67, 170–72
intercessory, 143–45
Priapus, 128
prison, 126
Promoter of the Faith (Devil's Advocate), 9, 17
psychoanalytic theory, 51, 52, 53, 136, 154, 163, 172
public health, 92

publication, medical, 12, 138–45, 165, 166
Puglia, 54, 75, 111–21, 184–85

Québec, 69–71, 149

Ravello, 123–25
Ravenna, 38, 103, 104
relics, 39, 45, 100, 104, 107, 109, 112, 116, 119, 124, 125, 127, 135, 158
religion
and medicine, 30, 37, 62, 63–64, 92, 93, 123, 137–45, 158, 161, 175
and science, 63–64, 90, 91, 129, 132, 141
See also Christianity; pagan religion
Renault, Chantal, 150, 152
research, 53, 58, 59, 61, 74, 80, 129–35, 147–48
funding of, 98
historical, 4, 16, 23, 28, 37, 54, 58, 62, 73, 93, 120, 130, 132–33, 135, 139, 166, 176
papers on, 52–54, 58–59, 61–63, 73, 92–95, 126
See also clinical trials; conferences; evidence; statistics; theories
Rey, Terry, 154
Riace, Italy, 86, 98, 106–9, 128, 129, 135
Riopel, Eulalie, 70
Risse, Guenter, 93
ritual, 17, 24, 64, 72, 152, 162, 166
Roberts, Leanne, 144
Rochester, Minn., 155
Roman Forum, 24, 31, 38, 43, 53
Romano, Terrie, 65, 67, 74
Rome, 19, 38–39, 41, 50, 117, 120, 129–35, 158, 160–63, 173
Romo, Ana Cecilia Rodríguez de, 89–92
Ronsard, Pierre de, 40
rules
for canonization, 5, 9, 11, 13, 15, 16, 17, 22, 26, 29, 30, 130
in hematology, 6, 7, 9, 10, 14, 29, 30

Saint Michael's College, Toronto, 47, 93, 94

saints, 21, 93–94, 141, 147, 152
  as healers, 31, 38, 45, 53, 165
  physician, 125, 132–33, 185–87
  role of, 21
  See also canonization; *and by specific name*

Salerno, 122–23, 124, 126

San Cosimato in Trastevere, Rome, 40, 133

San Cosmo Albanese, Italy, 71, 110–111, 114, 135

Sandor, Monica, 93

Santena, Turin, Italy, 128–29, 135

Santi Cosma e Damiano, Italy, 101

Sapena, Madre Sonia, 134

science. *See* religion and science

Sebastian, St., 25, 126

Segesta, Sicily, 104

September 11, 2001, 72, 101, 113, 116

Sferrocavallo, Sicily, 104, 129

Shein, Max and Rosita, 90, 101

shrines, 31, 38–40, 42, 44, 47, 53, 72, 69, 91, 100, 173

Sicily, 42, 46, 51, 73, 84, 101, 102, 103–6, 122, 132

Silano, Giulio, 94, 95, 129, 130, 136

Sisto, Giovanni, 111–17

skepticism, 13, 14, 29, 30, 46, 109, 167, 168, 169, 173, 177

slaves, 25, 152, 154

Slovenia, 40

sociological theory, 51–54, 89, 135, 154

sociology, 31, 58, 63, 64, 138, 152, 153

Sophronius, 34

Soto, Francisco de, 92

Spain, 40

spirituality, 23, 57, 85, 138, 141, 143, 145, 162, 163, 165, 166

St. Paul's University, Ottawa, 12

St. Peter's Basilica, 20, 25, 29

statistics, 13, 138, 142, 165, 169, 171, 173

statues
  in Europe, 40, 44, 100, 102, 104, 105, 106, 107, 109, 112, 114, 115, 116, 119, 127, 128, 129
  in Haïti, 83
  in Mexico, 91
  in Toronto, 46, 47, 48, 50, 155, 172, 173
  in the United States, 55–56, 68, 71, 75, 76, 77, 78, 79, 81, 82, 87, 88, 157

stethoscope, 65, 90, 100

Subiaco, Italy, 38

surgery, 21, 76, 79, 87, 88, 120, 123, 143, 155, 158

surveys, 64–69, 94, 136, 137, 138–45, 149, 165, 167
  results of, 83–89, 180–87
  See also interviews

Sutton's Law, 126

syncretism, 43, 44, 46, 150, 152, 153, 163

Syria, 33, 34, 39, 40

Taormina, Sicily, 104

technology, medical, 29, 138, 139, 155, 171, 173

Temkin, Owsei, 63

temples, 24, 36–37, 38, 41, 43, 44, 53, 88, 89, 98, 103, 104, 122, 128, 133, 135, 161

Theodore of Sykeon, St., 38

Theodoret of Cyr, 36, 73

theories, 51–52, 53, 58, 59, 65, 95, 121, 135–36, 154, 172–73

Thom, Robert, 147

Thunder Bay, Ontario, 3, 4

Toledo, Ohio, 40

Tomaselli, Dan, 77, 79

Toronto, 31–33, 46–51, 53, 54, 57, 58, 66–68, 69, 79–80, 83, 84, 86, 93–94, 117, 127, 135, 137, 145, 155, 172–73

Tours, France, 40

Toussaint, Yolette, 153–54

Townson, Andréa, 27–28
tribunal, ecclesiastical, 9, 11, 12, 13–15,
    16, 23
trulli, 112, 114, 116
Turkey, 33, 38
twins, 21, 24, 84–85, 87, 137
    as deities, 44–45, 51–52, 150, 154
    as healers, 39, 41, 150, 163, 172
Tyndall, John, 142, 144

Ukraine, 40, 73
Utica, New York, 48, 51, 54–57, 58,
    68–69, 84, 86, 89, 119, 127, 135, 147,
    172
Utti, Emmanuel, 147

Valilà, Renzo, 108–9, 128
Vatican, 7, 9, 10, 11, 23, 82, 95, 110,
    140
Vatican Archives, 16, 33, 129–35, 136, 167
Vatican Council, second, 43, 63
Vienna, 39

Vietnam, 89
Vitus, St., 125, 128
Vodou, 150–54
votives, 24, 40, 53, 89, 108, 109, 133, 158
    as paintings, 117, 120, 121

Washington, D.C., 82
weddings, 105, 127, 133, 161
wells, 100
Wetering, Ineke van, 63
witches, 61, 62
Wittmann, Anneliese, 40, 42, 105
Woestman, William H., 12, 14–15, 16
Wolfe, Jessica, 58, 73, 90, 91
Wolfe, Robert David, 4, 19, 20, 27, 58, 77,
    97, 98, 101, 117, 129, 130, 176
Woodward, Kenneth L., 17, 20, 23
World War II, 102

xenodochion, 38, 40

Zumárraga, Juan de, 92